Neuropsychology of Communication

Michela Balconi (Ed.)

Neuropsychology of Communication

Springer

Editor
Michela Balconi
Department of Psychology
Catholic University of Milan
Milan, Italy

This is a revised, enlarged and completely updated version of the Italian Edition published under the title
Neuropsicologia della comunicazione
edited by M. Balconi

ISBN 978-88-470-1583-8 ISBN 978-88-470-1584-5 (eBook)

DOI 10.1007/978-88-470-1584-5

Springer Milan Dordrecht Heidelberg London New York

Library of Congress Control Number: 2010925385

9 8 7 6 5 4 3 2 1

Cover design: Ikona S.r.l., Milan, Italy

Typesetting: Graphostudio, Milan, Italy

Springer-Verlag Italia S.r.l. – Via Decembrio 28 – I-20137 Milan
Springer is a part of Springer Science+Business Media (www.springer.com)

Preface

Not nothing
without you
but not the same
Erich Fried (1979)

Communication has become, in recent years, an autonomous field of theoretical reflection and a proficient research perspective, independent of the study of language and instead focused on the ensemble of competencies needed to produce and comprehend language. This independence is evidenced by the growing interest in the communicative process, addressed by disciplines such as the *social sciences*, with specific regard to social cognition, and *cognitive psychology*, which examines the role of cognitive representation in communication regulation as well as the metacognitive functions related to the self-other distinction in the regulation of conversational demands. The role and meaning of communication are determined by the confluence of multiple contributions, which share the condition of an agent who is interacting with other agents such that the representational systems and relational contexts among agents are mutually modified.

The link between communication and the field of neuropsychology is of particular interest. However, in its recent development, the latter has only marginally considered issues relevant to communicative processes, focusing instead on linguistic ones. Much remains to be learned regarding the pragmatic skills of communication, which thus far have been only partially explored from a neuropsychological perspective. Adequate theoretical and methodological tools with which to explore the complexity of communicative processes are still lacking. These processes include concepts such as the inferential model, mutual knowledge between speakers, and intentions decoding, and require the use of sophisticated instruments able to represent interpersonal contexts, the realm where communication operates. The need to distinguish between "closed" (within speakers' minds) and "open" and "acted" highlights the importance of novel research domains, such as the newly developed field of neuropragmatics.

A neuropsychologically based understanding of communication is likely to remain a challenge rather than an ultimately reached goal. Many aspects of communication have yet to be adequately explored, for example, non-verbal components, which include the vocal features and gestural elements of the communicative act.

Other aspects, such as the study of mimic and facial expressions, are more advanced, especially with respect to emotion communication. Another and even more difficult goal is the integration of different indices of analysis, i.e., behavioral, psychophysiological, and neuropsychological measures, in order to explain the contribution of old and new theoretical models and to confirm or, in some cases, reject previously consolidated perspectives.

This book considers these and other important topics in communication. Section I, *The Neuropsychology of Language and Communication*, provides an anatomic-functional perspective. Its four chapters review the contributions made to the study of language, linguistic functions, and communication by the neuropsychological approach. The first chapter considers the neuropsychology of language and communication; specifically, developments in the field over the last decade and the sub-specialties of neurolinguistics and neuropragmatics. Particular attention is paid to knowledge gained through the latter and through social neuroscience. Methodological and technical advances are explored in Chapter 2, which reviews the main and more recent techniques of analysis: neuroimaging (fMRI, PET), magnetic supports (TMS, MEG), and electrophysiological measures (ERPs). The significance of these new technologies in the study of communication is the topic of Chapter 3, which describes the applications of transcranial magnetic stimulation in the study of linguistic and communicative competences. This non-invasive tool allows investigation of the neuronal basis of language in normal subjects. Chapter 4 explores the processes underlying language comprehension, both in the visual modality of reading and in the auditory modality of listening, by focusing on the main stages of linguistic information processing, from the sensory to the symbolic level.

The book's second section, *Neuropragmatics. Psychophysiological, Neuropsychological and Cognitive Correlates*, covers the new discipline of neuropragmatics, with specific attention paid to the relationship between theoretical models, such as pragmatic representation of the speech act, and neural correlates underlying the associated processes. Chapter 5 investigates these topics further in terms of the significance of the relationship between the brain structures, functions, and mental processes involved in language use. Metaphors, idioms, general non-compositional strings, and irony are considered through the application of different neuropsychological methodologies. In Chapter 6, "idiomatic" and "iconic" meanings are analyzed; the main experimental paradigms used are briefly reported and insights gained from studies on patients with focal brain damage are discussed. The chapter closes with a brief mention of idiomatic comprehension in Alzheimer's disease and what has been learned in investigations of a psychiatric population (schizophrenics). Chapter 7 considers the semantic and iconic correlates of idioms, examining the role of anticipatory mechanisms in the comprehension of idiomatic expressions. These multiword strings are characterized by the fact that their meaning is conventionalized and their constituents are bound together in a predefined order. In Chapter 8, which concludes section, new insights into the neurophysiological mechanisms responsible for linguistic processing are presented, including selected examples of the "neurobiological" approach to syntactic rule acquisition, semantic representation, and speech perception/production.

The important role of intentions in communication and the contribution of different communicative systems (such as nonverbal components) are analyzed in the third section of the book, *From Intentions to Nonverbal Communication*. The relationship between intentionality and communicative intentions is discussed in Chapter 9, which highlights the role of consciousness and working memory in communication and considers action strategy, inferential abilities, and mentalization competencies. The contribution of social neuroscience is recognized, especially in exploring the relation between meta-cognition and communication skills. Chapter 10 introduces the topic of nonverbal communication. Neuropsychological studies have underlined the significant presence of distinct brain correlates assigned to analyze the facial expression of emotion and have distinguished the contributions of the two hemispheres in comprehending the emotional face, as a function of emotion type (positive vs. negative) and specific tasks (comprehending vs. producing facial expressions). In the last chapter (Chapter 11), the nonverbal communication of emotions is assessed, with specific regard to the brain correlates of attitude and personality. The role that temperament plays in influencing cortical responses to mimic components is analyzed, taking into account subjective sensitivity to environmental emotional cues by using the BIS/BAS model (behavioral inhibition vs. activation system).

This book is intended as an important resource for researchers and professionals in the field of communication. Moreover, I hope that the book's readers are able to improve and expand their communicative skills, by exploring the direct relationship between brain and communication.

Special thanks are extended to my husband, with whom I have a highly valued communicative relationship.

The volume was partially funded by the Catholic University of Milan (D3.1. 2008).

Milan, June 2010 **Michela Balconi**

Contents

List of Contributors

Simona Amenta
Department of Psychology
Catholic University of Milan
Milan, Italy

Michela Balconi
Department of Psychology
Catholic University of Milan
Milan, Italy

Cristina Cacciari
Department of Biomedical Sciences
University of Modena and Reggio Emilia
Modena, Italy

Paolo Canal
Department of Biomedical Sciences
University of Modena and Reggio Emilia
Modena, Italy

Stefano F. Cappa
Vita-Salute San Raffaele University
and Division of Neuroscience
San Raffaele Scientific Institute
Milan, Italy

Maria Cotelli
Cognitive Neuroscience Section
IRCCS San Giovanni di Dio Fatebenefratelli
Brescia, Italy

Alice Mado Proverbio
Department of Psychology
University of Milano-Bicocca
Milan, Italy

Rosa Manenti
Cognitive Neuroscience Section
IRCCS San Giovanni di Dio
Fatebenefratelli
Brescia, Italy

Carlo Miniussi
Department of Biomedical Sciences
and Biotechnologies
National Institute of Neuroscience
University of Brescia
Brescia, Italy
Cognitive Neuroscience Section
IRCCS San Giovanni di Dio Fatebenefratelli
Brescia, Italy

Nicola Molinaro
Basque Center on Cognition,
Brain and Language
Donostia-San Sebastián, Spain

Costanza Papagno
Department of Psychology
University of Milano-Bicocca
Milan, Italy

Francesco Vespignani
Department of Cognitive and
Education Sciences
University of Trento
Rovereto (TN), Italy

Alberto Zani
CNR - Institute of Molecular Bioimaging
and Physiology
Segrate (MI), Italy

Section I
The Neuropsychology of Language and Communication

Biological Basis of Linguistic and Communicative Systems: From Neurolinguistics to Neuropragmatics

1

M. Balconi

1.1
Introduction: Neuropsychology for Language and Communication

Humans characterize themselves by their ability to build instruments, among which language is the most relevant. Language is used in order to communicate thoughts and feelings to other individuals through the systematic combination of sounds, gestures, and symbols. This ability allows humans to reach other humans from a distance, both temporal and spatial. Moreover, language shapes the social structure of humans and is the most powerful medium to convey cognitive and emotional states and to give form to interpersonal relationships. All these attributes define and constitute our linguistic and communicative systems.

Language comprehension requires specific competencies, such as the ability of choosing, at different levels, particular structures and configurations among a continuous flow of visual and acoustic inputs [1, 2]. Phonemes, morphemes, syllables, words, sentences, discourse, and, on a higher level, general conceptual structures are constructed starting from simple sensorial signals. Those levels are organized in flexible ways and individuals have the skill to produce and construct new sound strings or signs that have never been produced or heard before. In addition, speakers are not only able to understand linguistic stimuli, they are also capable of performing systematic changes in vocal traits and the motor system, so as to reach a more complex verbal and non-verbal communication, by converting concepts into a precise sequence of motor commands.

Recently, there has been a growing interest in the relations between linguistic and communicative processes and the underlying cortical structures supporting them. Specifically, questions have been formulated regarding the nature of the relation

M. Balconi (✉)
Department of Psychology, Catholic University of Milan, Milan, Italy

1

between linguistic and communicative components and neuropsychology. Furthermore, the study of neurophysiological processes of language production and comprehension has generated new questions on how brain structure and plasticity can mediate linguistic flexibility. Which cortical and sub-cortical areas are majorly involved in communicative process and which function do they have? How and in which temporal order are they activated in the different steps of language and communication?

Generally, neuropsychological data allow testing of the psychological plausibility of the different constructs proposed by the principal psycholinguistic models (*neurolinguistics*) [3]. For instance, psycholinguistics has hypothesized the existence of a structured mental lexicon whose components mediate the phonological, orthographic, morphologic, and semantic traits of words [4]. How can we collect evidence endorsing or refuting the existence of such representational levels and their organization in the brain? Neuropsychological data allow the formulation of theories describing how different representations are used during language production and comprehension. Some models, for instance, have proposed that particular subprocesses are instantiated in highly specialized and independent modules [5, 6]. These models assume that specific cortical areas are dedicated to the elaboration of different types of representations, that they have a reduced influence on one another, and that they are activated in a precise temporal sequence (e.g., syntactic precedes semantic which precedes pragmatic processes) [7, 8]. By contrast, according to interactive models, lower elaboration levels are not independent from higher processes as they interact continuously [9].

Another open issue is related to how linguistic structure derives from neurobiological language-specific processes, or how linguistic processes are conditioned by general cognitive constraints, such as attentive resource availability or working memory functioning. In other words, neurobiological data allow us not only to understand the nature of linguistic representations and processes, but also to explain how language develops and how it can be compromised in cases of trauma and deficits [10, 11]. Generally, it is necessary to define which factors affect brain functioning and how those factors can influence linguistic and communicative functions.

Finally, are there specific functions for the *language in use*; that is, for pragmatic functions which confer meaning on communicative messages in real and "contextualized" contexts? The study of pragmatic aspects of communication through the neuropsychological approach (*neuropragmatics*, see Par. 1.6) has opened up new perspectives on how the communicative process takes place, ensuring the mutual exchange of shared meanings within conversational contexts [12, 13].

At this point, it is necessary to introduce a few relevant distinctions, first of all by highlighting the reasons accounting for the dual dichotomy between *linguistic functions* and *communicative functions* on one side, and between the ability to *produce* and to *comprehend* meanings on the other. The first proposed distinction aims to individuate distinctive components of processes that have been investigated independently from each other, in order to integrate them in a global representation. The nature of the distinction *language vs communication* is, in fact, fictitious, since language and communication are indeed contiguous levels of a global process oriented to the transmission of meanings between speakers. Distinguishing an abstract language, whose proprieties are defined regardless of context, is indeed of interest only in theoretical studies, but it does not match actual conditions of use. Any communicative act is intentional and it is performed to achieve the mutual exchange and comprehension of meanings. Therefore, language is instrumental for a wider communicative process, which implies the presence, actual or virtual, of two or more interacting individuals in a given context.

As regards the second proposed dichotomy, it is necessary to consider the complexity of the communicative act, which consists in the dual task of elaborating meanings in order to transmit (output process) and receive (incoming process) them. It is therefore necessary to distinguish between production and comprehension, as aspects which are intertwined but independent from one another. In fact, also on the neuropsychological level, deficits in production do not imply necessarily deficits in comprehension, and vice versa [14-16].

By adopting the cognitive neuropsychology perspective, in this chapter we focus on both linguistic and communicative processes. We discuss competencies required to produce and understand communicative messages and the functioning of the cognitive and neural systems underneath those functions. The paragraph following this Introduction presents the state of the art of the structural and anatomic components underlying language and communication. The next paragraph focuses on the principal linguistic functions and systems (morphologic, syntactic, semantic, and conceptual). Finally, the last paragraph is dedicated to communicative components, with particular attention paid to the pragmatic dimension (prosody, discourse, conversation, and social competences). We consider "pragmatics" in a broader sense (beyond the boundaries suggested by linguistic pragmatics and cognitive neuropragmatics [17, 18]), shifting the focus from communicative products (e.g., ironic communication or discourse properties) to cognitive processes activated in communication and their intrinsic characteristics.

1.2 Properties and Functions of Linguistic and Communicative Processes

Here, we focus on three features that characterize the linguistic and communication domains: the *structural* and *functional multiplicity* of systems underlying language and communication; the *multi-componentiality* of those systems, particularly related to non-verbal components; and their intrinsic *dynamism*.

With regard to structural multiplicity, it is necessary to point out that the neurophysiological components underlying language and communication are heterogeneous. This heterogeneity refers specifically to the variety of cortical and sub-cortical structures intervening in the regulation of different linguistic and communicative functions [19]. Throughout the years, different models have tried to define the brain map of the principal mechanisms involved in language and communication production and comprehension. At present, the data favor the involvement of a multiplicity of structures, and thus both different typologies of functional units (see below) and the distinction between production and comprehension [20]. Although it is still not possible to define a one-to-one map tracing a clear correspondence between specific processes and specific brain structures, in many cases it has been possible to individuate the contribution of precise cortical and sub-cortical components related to the principal communicative functions. It is worth noting that "brain maps" do not refer to circumscribed brain areas, since it is preferable to use distributed models as a reference [21].

The functional multiplicity of linguistic and communicative processes refers to a *hierarchy of interconnected functions*. The main components mainly ascribed to linguistic functions are:

1. *phonologic components*: phonemes, their functions, and the rules that govern their organization;
2. *morphology* (including the smallest meaningful units of a language, which could also be mere phonemes): the form of words and related variations connected with their meanings and functions;
3. *lexicon*: word level (the combination of phonemes that results in a conceptual meaning);
4. *syntax*: comprising basic principles that are finalized to associate words in order to construct syntagms (syntactic strings of words that constitute the phrase basic units), phrases, and sentences;
5. *semantics*: the meaning of the words and sentences.

Superordinate to the components listed above, *grammar* concerns rules applied to linguistic constituents in order to regulate language use. Finally, *pragmatics* deals with meanings in context and considers language as a system oriented to "communicate messages," often going beyond "what is said" [22, 23].

The pragmatic level is generally identified as "what is meant" by the speaker and it is related to communicative functions and competences (see Par. 1.5). Without adopting a componential perspective [24], pragmatics would be nonetheless considered as a superordinate level, as it implies a broader representational level than levels typically referring to basic linguistic functions [25]. In fact, the pragmatic level uses linguistic and non-linguistic (non-verbal) components to communicate meaning. These components refer basically to the extra-linguistic level, which is mainly dedicated to express speakers' intentions, goals, thoughts, and emotions. Compared to the generic finality of constructing meanings, mainly attributed to language, pragmatics accomplishes the task of regulating the communicative exchange, based on the sharing of intentional levels. Through pragmatics, the transmission of meanings between individuals is assured, relationships are regulated, and the psychological boundaries of interactions are defined.

With regard to cognitive competencies required by the pragmatic level, it is necessary to refer to *inferential competencies* (ostensive-inferential, following the Sperber and Wilson model [25]), *mental states attribution* (generally considered under the theory of mind model [26]), *social functions* definition [27, 28], and *mutual exchange regulation* [29]. The role of context is particularly relevant, especially with regards to the cognitive and emotional components framing communicative interaction [30].

In particular, we aim to overcome the limits of cognitive pragmatics and neuropragmatics, which are focused in some cases on interactive [31] and strictly cognitive aspects of communication (with particular references to mental models and script theories) [32, 33], in order to define the domains of *cognitive*, *communicative*, and *relational* competencies, which jointly act to enable the construction, transmission, and comprehension of meanings. Therefore, pragmatics is intended here not only as the study of "what is meant in context," but also must take into account a broad range of processes oriented to the transmission of meanings among individuals in real situations, thus requiring general social competencies (*social cognition*) [34]. The principal domains involving pragmatics abilities are:

1. *vocal non-verbal components*, including prosodic functions in general and emotional prosody in particular, whose deficits have been investigated by clinical neuropragmatics [35];
2. *linguistic pragmatic functions*, such as figurative language (e.g., idioms, metaphors, irony), and indirect speech acts in general [36-38];
3. *discourse* and *conversation*, which are the domain of *discourse pragmatics* [39, 40];
4. *social cognition competencies*, which are intended as the ensemble of competencies that rule the relations between individuals and their environment [34].

The last category can be viewed as transversal, since all pragmatic phenomena are framed by the social context of the interaction.

From what has been said so far, it appears that communication is a multi-component process, since it employs multiple communicative channels in order to transmit meanings; not only verbal components, but also gestural and mimic elements participate in communication. In particular, non-verbal components are specific to pragmatic functions even if they perform linguistic functions as well (see Chapter 8). Communication multi-componentiality raises a question about the existence of distinctive neuropsychological correlates specific for different systems and about the synchronization of these different components [41, 42].

A last consideration addresses the *dynamic nature* of language and communication, since both are developing functions within a process that involves the *negotiation* and *syntonization* of meanings [43]. Recently, pragmatics studies on interactive processes have focused on the diachronicity of communication and its development throughout the interaction [44]. Generally, it is necessary to underline that linguistic and communicative competencies presuppose a progressive learning and evolution that take place throughout development, on both the phylogenetic and the ontogenetic level, in which a continuous modification of communicative and linguistic competencies occurs.

1.3 Anatomic-structural Models of Language Functioning

1.3.1 Classical Models

Different models have tried to define the contributions of the anatomic structures supporting human linguistic competencies, with evidence for either a "focal" (cortical module models) or a "distributed" (cortical network models) representation of these components [5, 45]. Notwithstanding the heterogeneity of the available data, the majority of authors agree on two main points: (1) the *left hemisphere* is dominant for language and (2) the areas of *Broca* and *Wernicke* have a prominent role in, respectively, the *production* and *understanding* of language. Here we consider both assumptions, highlighting their heuristic functions in language processing analysis as well as pointing out several critical issues.

Concerning the first assumption, there is a general agreement about differences between the two hemispheres regarding both the anatomic (cytoarchitecture) and functional levels. Left brain dominance has been proved not only through structural analyses, but also through electrophysiological measurements. Cortical event-related potentials (ERPs, see Chaps. 2 and 4) have provided evidence of the augmented sensitivity of the left hemisphere for language, beginning at birth [46]. Clinical studies have produced analogous data on patients with split-brain syndrome and those who are commissurotomized (corpus callosum severance) [47]. Similarly, using the dichotic listening procedure (giving two slightly different acoustic stimuli, one to the left ear and the other to the right ear) on healthy subjects, a functionally different response of the two hemispheres in linguistic tasks has been observed [48].

It is now necessary to question the origins of hemispheric lateralization: does it precede or follow the development of language abilities? The theory of *brain structure equipotentiality* assumes that lateralization is a consequence of linguistic development. However, this hypothesis cannot explain, on either the ontogenetic or the phylogenetic level, the reasons for the evolutionary selection of the right hemisphere and the subsequent advantages for human species. Moreover, language areas appear to be anatomically and functionally asymmetric well before the development of language, as research on the temporal planum, localized in proximity to the primary auditory cortex (near the Wernicke area), has evidenced. Hemispheric asymmetry is already evident at the 31st week of gestation and is strictly connected to individual handedness: 96% of right-handed individuals show a greater hemispheric specialization (a more extended temporal planum) compared to 70% of left-handed individuals. Another distinction concerns the corpus callosum, which connects the hemispheres and therefore is responsible for the transmission of information arriving from opposite body parts. A difference in the isthmus size has been observed that is inversely proportional to the temporal planum size, with a greater extension of the isthmus of the corpus callosum potentially related to a decreased extension of the temporal planum, with a subsequent reduced asymmetry for linguistic functions [49].

As far as the Broca/Wernicke dichotomy is concerned, the largely accredited Wernicke-Geschwind model assumes that specific brain regions and their connections are responsible for the representation of linguistic functions. The model suggests that distinct anatomic components perform specific input-output functions for the production and comprehension of language; therefore, damage to these areas can result in a specific deficit of the related cognitive and linguistic abilities. Circumscribed lesions to perisylvian area usually produce deficits limited to certain linguistic functions (*aphasic syndromes*): for example, *production aphasia* (or motor aphasia) results from lesions in Broca's region, while lesions to Wernicke's area produce *comprehension aphasia*. Broca's area, localized close to the inferior motor cortex (prefrontal gyrus), controls language production and the motor commands necessary for the articulation of words, facial mimic, and phonation. Compromise of this region results in an impaired ability to express words but with preserved phonatory abilities. Conversely, Wernicke's area, located within the posterior section of the superior temporal gyrus, has a predominant role in verbal language comprehension processes. Damage to this area results in disfluent oral production (jargon-like) accompanied by the appearance of neologisms. The location and extent of Broca's and Wernicke's areas are shown in Figure 1.1.

The Wernicke-Geschwind model predicts that oral language reaches the auditory cortex but if Wernicke's area is lesioned it is not activated, thus impairing oral comprehension. If the area involved by the lesion extends beyond Wernicke's region and includes areas that cause the deterioration of visual input elaboration, then deficits in both oral and written language comprehension can occur. By contrast, lesions to Broca's area cause a severe alteration of discourse production, since the motor scheme for sound emission and language structure is not transmitted to the motor cortex. Finally, lesions to the arcuate fasciculus disrupt the connection between Broca's and Wernicke's areas, thus causing alteration of discourse flow. In particular, it would not be possible through feedback circuits for auditory afferences to reach Broca's area and for information relative to language production to be re-transmitted to regions involved with comprehension [49].

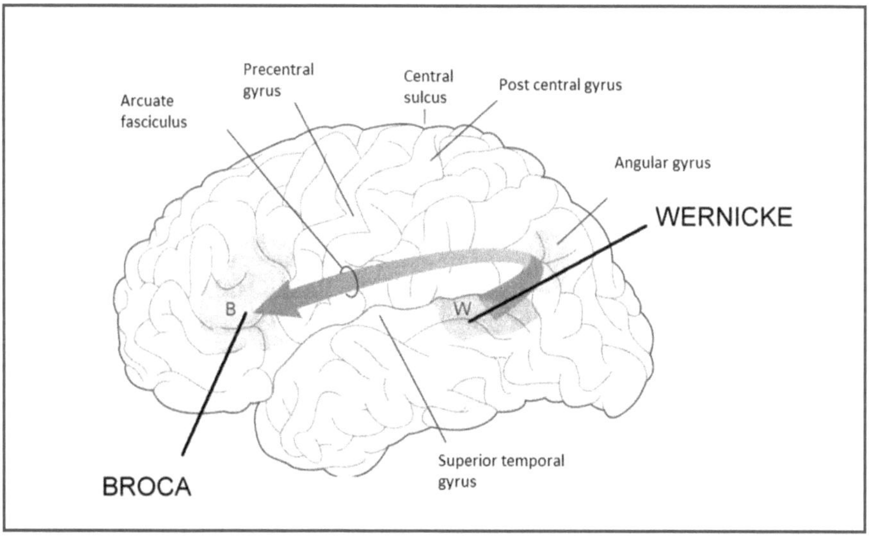

Fig 1.1 Representation of Broca's and Wernicke's areas and their connections

1

1.3.2 Recent Acquisitions: Sub-cortical Systems and Interface Areas

The specificity of Broca's and Wernicke's areas for language production and understanding has been questioned by modern neurolinguistics [50], due to the introduction of advanced neuroimaging techniques. In fact, lesion studies, such as those that led to formulation of the Wernicke-Geschwind model, could not account for individual differences in brain organization and re-organization following a traumatic event.

Recent empirical findings led to the inclusion of other neural systems in addition to the traditional areas. Thus, the left temporal regions, left prefrontal cortex, thalamus, and supplementary motor area have been shown to be involved in language processes [51]. A crucial role was recently attributed to sub-cortical structures, such as the left thalamus, left caudate nucleus, and contiguous white matter. In particular, the left caudate nucleus is considered to be crucial for the integration of auditory and motor representation, both of which are necessary for language processing. In fact, lesions to this system result in the alteration of auditory comprehension [52]. The thalamus seems to have a crucial, although supportive, role in language processing since it increases the efficacy of linguistic production.

Limitations to the traditional model have also been detailed in recent studies within the cognitive sciences, showing that not all acoustic afferences are elaborated along the same paths; rather, meaningful and meaningless sounds seem to be elaborated independently. In other words, different neural paths are thought to elaborate general expressive sound units and the morphemic units that retain a semantic content. Moreover, processes of language comprehension and production (written and oral) seem to include a greater number of systems than hypothesized by the Wernicke-Geschwind model.

Analyses of patients who underwent surgical treatment for epilepsy suggested the existence of different response systems for different typologies of linguistic stimuli [53]. Furthermore, some cells that appear to be highly activated in response to linguistic process are located bilaterally in the medial portion of the superior temporal gyrus, thus questioning left hemispheric dominance for language production and comprehension. Recently, patients with split-brain syndrome were shown to be able to recognize and discriminate sounds [54] and syntactically simple sentences [55]. Those data suggest that the language comprehension system can be organized bilaterally. At the same time, a functional magnetic resonance imaging (fMRI) study registered the contribution of the left superior posterior temporal region in language production tasks (object naming) [56]. Finally, behavioral studies have shown a tight correlation between production and comprehension processes. Experimental studies demonstrated a reduction of the verbal transformation effect (the incorrect perception of phonemes following the repeated presentation of a word) [57] when subjects were asked to perform verbal production (also sub-vocalic). These data suggest that production and comprehension processes share distinct units.

Therefore, taken together, the data indicate that a model can be formulated that accounts for the existence of broad interface zones [58, 59] or intermediate representational levels [60-62] (Fig. 1.2). This model posits a strong interdependence between

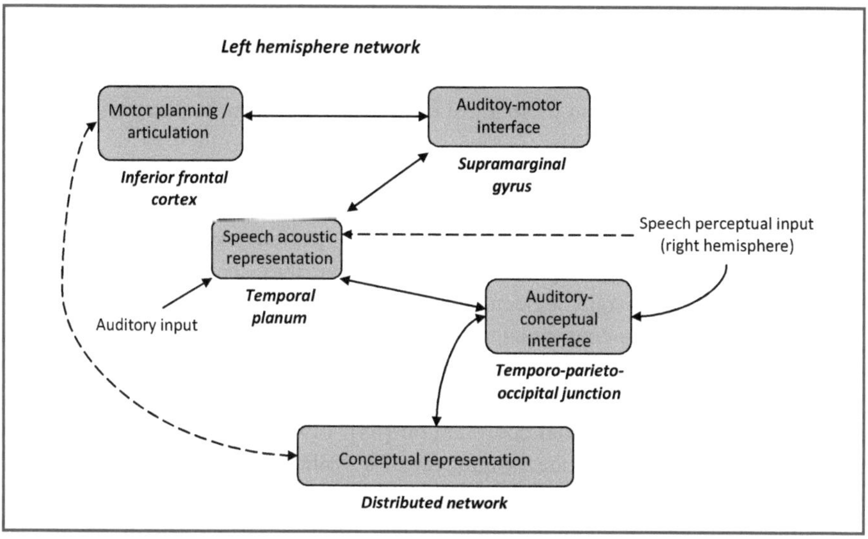

Fig. 1.2 Neuroanatomic model of the language network, showing the relevance of the areas of interface between the left and right brain

the right and left hemispheres, with the former assuming perceptive processes that transmit inputs to auditory-conceptual interface systems within the left hemisphere. Auditory-based interface systems would interfere with conceptual and frontal motor systems through a second auditory motor interface area, located in the inferior parietal lobe. Similar to previous models [63], this model presupposes a direct link between conceptual representation and frontal lobe systems. Given the highly distributed nature of conceptual representation, it is possible to hypothesize a convergence of multiple inputs in frontal cortex interface zones [58, 59], evidenced, for example, by the role of some regions of the left inferior temporal lobe in accessing conceptual/lexical representations of objects in language production [64].

1.4 The Contribution of Neurolinguistics

1.4.1 Language Production and Comprehension Processes: Cognitive Models

A thorough neuropsychological analysis of linguistic processes should also include a description of the principal linguistic functions, i.e., the ability to produce, understand, and coordinate phonologic, syntactic, and semantic structures [1]. Those functions depend upon a variety of representational systems, which include linguistic information elaboration systems, non-verbal information decoding systems, and conceptual elaboration devices.

1

Modern neurolinguistics explicitly aims to dissect and analyze linguistic mechanisms, based on the assumption that the mental processes underlying linguistic functions are separable and that it is possible to define the complex architecture of linguistic systems starting from its smallest elementary unit, that is, phonetic representation.

The model proposed by Levelt [61] allows analysis of the complexity of the operations and cognitive processes involved in message production (top-down) and comprehension (bottom-up). As shown in Figure 1.3, production and comprehension comprise a multiplicity of cognitive units; moreover, they share elaboration levels, such as phonology, prosody, lexicon, syntax, and the message level, relative to discourse structure and the conceptual system. Both systems appear to be characterized by two principal elaboration flows: *lexical production/decoding* and *phrasal structure construction/re-construction*. The distinction between these functions poses a problem regarding their mutual coordination [65]. Lexical representation processes seem to be concurrent with the assignment of a syntactic structure to the string of words composing a sentence, following an incremental and sequential principle. Therefore, in sentence comprehension, lexical form is assimilated by the phrase structure, which is defined by the contribution of the prosodic level. Furthermore, as shown in Figure 1.3, lexical assignment, preceded by acoustic and phonetic elaboration, does not directly depend upon word meaning, as it is instead controlled by lemmas

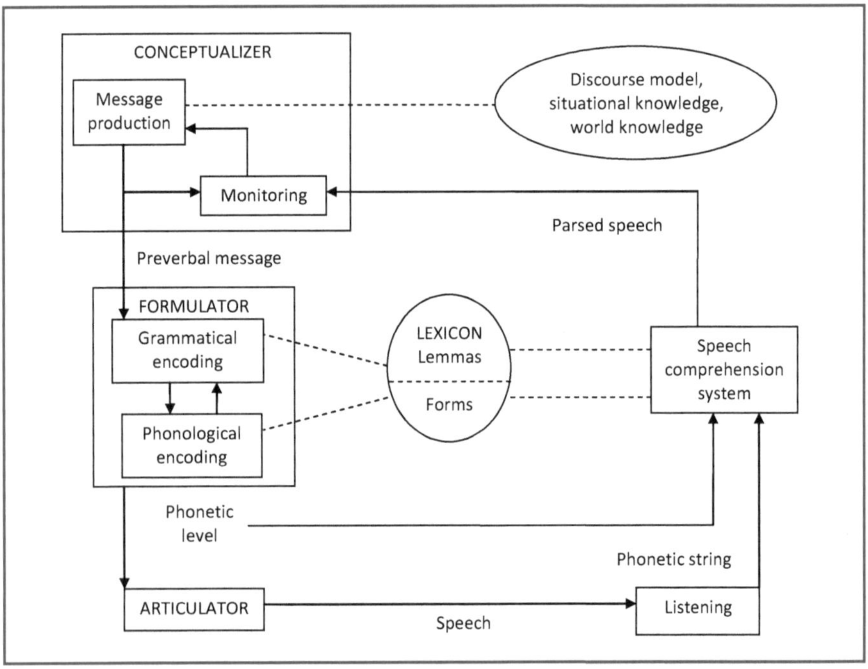

Fig. 1.3. Language production and comprehension. (Modified from Levelt [90])

that guide its formal properties. The next phase, denominated parsing, implies the assignment of structural-syntactic components, such as thematic role definition, predication, and co-reference functions.

The top-down process of production involves the same sequence of events, but in reverse order: syntactic construction precedes the lemmas guiding phonologic attribution and the assimilation of the formal structure established by these lemmas into the prosodic and phrasal structure, while articulation ends the sequence.

The principle of independence and autonomy of these levels (*functional modularity*) represents the foundation of the entire process of organization, although it is necessary that the different levels are activated simultaneously and that they are able to interact with each other in order to perform the on-line production/comprehension of messages. Examples of the independence and interaction of representational systems and functions are provided below.

1.4.2 Functional Modularity of Language and Independence of Conceptual, Syntactic, and Semantic Representation Systems

Language modularity, intended as the ensemble of different processes and cognitive operations, has been analyzed extensively through a variety of methodologies (for a review, see [66]). In particular, the hypothesis of the functional organization of language predicts that three main autonomous systems are involved in linguistic representations: a *conceptual system* (representation of contents/concepts), a *structural system* (representation of words functions and phrase structure), and *semantic system* (representation of the global meaning of the message). The modality proposed by this hypothesis is incremental. Levelt [8] suggested that a functional incremental model governs the construction of messages, including meta-cognitive operations such as *macroplanning* and *microplanning*. Both levels can be further divided into specific operations (e.g., conceptual system activation during macroplanning, or morphophonologic encoding during microplanning). Macroplanning deals specifically with what the speaker wants to communicate, and thus the mental model formulation about the self and others; discourse structure definition and communication monitoring are also operations performed by macroplanning. The speaker's message generally aims to influence the interlocutor's mental models: therefore, to be successful, message construction requires and involves social competencies and common ground. Message construction is therefore the result of complex cognitive operations and, as such, it appears to be mainly conceptual. Microplanning, by contrast, deals with the organization of linguistic units into a coherent representation of the message: it operates from preverbal conceptual representations to verbal messages. Each unit should be transposed into a specific format in order to be verbally formulated. The phrase structure defined by this level should include semantic and functional relations that can be expressed through language.

The assumptions underlying this model provide relevant theoretical foundations for those who agree on a functional organization of cortical structure. Traditional

1

psycholinguistic models, for instance, suggest the existence of separated neural structures as well as functional devices, which are responsible for performing semantic and conceptual processes, on the one hand, and for lexical form representation, on the other [67]. Experimental evidence has shown that corresponding to a preserved ability to recognize the lexical form of words is an inability to attribute the correct meaning to lexemes. Further evidence of the independence of these two representational levels is provided by the observation of specific deficits relative to conceptual categories of words (e.g., abstract/concrete or animate/inanimate). There are also individuals who are not able to recognize specific grammatical categories (e.g., nouns, verbs, prepositions), notwithstanding the correct comprehension of a given lexeme's meaning.

Frazier [68] proposed a model that explained the dissociation between syntactic and conceptual systems. A syntactic system can be defined as the ensemble of the functional categories of words and their relations (e.g., thematic roles, modifiers); these categories are hierarchically organized. As noted above, the conceptual system is formed by interrelated representations of knowledge about the world and its physical and non-physical objects. Linguistic, contextual, and pragmatic knowledge are also represented within the conceptual system, but the abilities to form concepts and to construct complex linguistic structure appear to be dissociated. In fact, focal lesions impairing the conceptual system are compatible with a preserved linguistic functioning of the morphologic and syntactic levels; thus, the lack of general representational ability is not linked to the ability to form and recognize a syntactically correct structure.

The syntactic system appears to be independent also with respect to semantics [69]. Neuroimaging data have shown different brain areas active in semantic and syntactic tasks. Furthermore, deficits in the semantic system, such as those in semantic dementia, are associated with lesions to the superior temporal lobe and can coexist with unaltered phonological and syntactic functions [67]. This dissociation is supported also by electrophysiological data. ERP studies have provided evidence in favor of distinct neural patterns for the elaboration of semantic and syntactic information [70-72]. In particular, semantic interpretation is indexed by the *N400* effect, which is temporally and spatially distinct from a syntactic elaboration index, i.e., the *P600* effect (see Chapter 4). It is necessary to note, however, that empirical studies have recently evidenced an interaction between these systems which allows the construction of meaningful sentences (see [67] for a review).

Finally, a dissociation has been noted between semantic and conceptual meanings, as a function of representational modalities. Word meaning is in fact represented within the semantic system. The latter is distinct from the conceptual system as it is responsible for encoding linguistically relevant aspects of a more general world knowledge, represented by the conceptual system [73]. The coincidence between the two systems, as proposed by Jackendoff [2], cannot, in fact, account for certain cognitive and linguistic phenomena, such as *conceptual ignorance* (individuals who can use a word in a semantically correct meaning without knowing its corresponding conceptual equivalent) or polysemy. Moreover, the existence of a unique or multiple semantic system that is dependent on the information-encoding modality is a current issue of discussion. Some authors suggest that the semantic system is based on a propositional format and, therefore, it is accessed by information from different sensorial channels [61]. However, according to other models [2], semantic representation is mediated by the perceptual modality of the input (*representational multimodality*).

1.5 Neuropsychology of Superior Communicative Functions: Neuropragmatics

Communication involves more than the mere ability to construct correct sentences and to decode their contents. The ability to perform a successful communicative act also implies specific assumptions about the symbolic properties of communication [74], starting from the ability to manipulate complex units, elaborate and comprehend complex inferential levels [22, 25], and develop and share a mutual system of rules in order to regulate communicative exchange [75]. In particular, it is necessary to plan the communicative act, to organize its elements into a coherent and cohesive discourse, while taking the context of the interaction into account [76]. Thus, an analysis of communicative competence should also address the issue of pragmatic functions and the ability to organize and integrate verbal and non-verbal signals [77]. Moreover, it is necessary to consider the specific cognitive competencies that allow individuals to communicate, that is, the ability to form, comprehend, and reflect on mental states (meta-cognition) [34], social cognition [27], and processes of intentionalization and re-intentionalization [78, 79] (see Chapter 9).

Here, communication is defined as an interactive process and, on a cognitive level, as an inferential process. In the following, we focus on the meta-cognitive and relational competencies that mediate the production and comprehension of language within communicative interactions. It should be noted that the study of communication has often been replaced with the study of language, as an abstract ability. This, in turn, has generated a distinction between the analysis of *language* and the analysis of the *use of language*. Actually, according to the communicative perspective, it is not possible to understand language independently from the cognitive, emotional, and relational components involved in the process. In other words, it is not possible to disregard the pragmatic context when we understand a specific meaning.

The introduction of advanced research methods into the field of neuropsychology has allowed investigation of the cortical contribution to the production/comprehension of meaning within a specific context, by focusing on the pragmatic aspects of communication (*neuropragmatics*). Neuropragmatics originated from an interaction between the different theoretical and experimental approaches that define its main branches: *experimental neuropragmatics* (the implementation of neuropsychological, psycholinguistic, and neurolinguistic methodologies and theoretical frameworks in the study of communicative competence) [12], *cognitive neuropragmatics* (the application of cognitive models to the study of pragmatics), and *clinical neuropragmatics* (the study of deficits of pragmatic functions) [80].

More recently, neuropragmatics has expanded to include the acquisition and functions of social cognitive competencies and the development of meta-representational abilities in communication [28]. The necessity to analyze communicative processes *during* communicative interactions has been pointed out, as it allows consideration of the influence of relational dynamics on the neuropsychological level. In other words, it is necessary to focus on the different brain structures and functional components activated by different processes involved in communication, such as emotional components, intentional levels, and relational elements. The analysis of brain networks involved in communication allows the on-line examination of specific processes, thus integrating linguistic and non-linguistic components, such as the motor activity finalized to regulate non-verbal communication, working memory contribution to the activity of regulation and synchronization of different systems and processes, and attention and intentionality in planning the communicative act [81].

From a bottom-up perspective, that is, from the observation of communicative dynamics to the analyses of involved processes, it is possible to investigate interactions among the linguistic, visual/acoustic, and motor systems [82]. For instance, there is a difference relating to the elaboration of phonological units, depending on the presence or absence of visual stimuli that reproduce the motor act for phonemic articulation [83]. Moreover, motor representation is crucial in non-verbal communication, in which specific cortical systems are activated [84]. The relation between action and communication has been reinforced by evidence indicating a strong link between communication and motor systems. In general, gestural activity during discourse production improves mnestic performance [85], while conversation and interactions can be seen as a progressive process of accommodation between the interlocutor's verbal and non-verbal systems.

In the following, the main components involved in linguistic processes within interactive contexts is described, from the microcommunicative units related to the vocal system, to the sentence unit that produces different typologies of communicative acts, to the macrocommunicative elements that refer mostly to discourse and conversation.

1.5.1 Paralinguistic Components

Paralinguistic aspects of communication include prosodic and suprasegmental structure of messages [86]. In this paragraph, we focus especially on pragmatic functions reached through the prosodic system, with particular attention paid to affective features.

1.5.1.1 Prosodic System

The prosodic system is a constituent of the wider paralinguistic system and performs a crucial role in the organization of communication and discourse functions. As a suprasegmental component, prosody connotes words [87] through the modulation of acoustic parameters such as intonation, pitch, volume, stress, and rhythm. Trager [88] introduced a specific classification of vocal non-linguistic components, paralanguage, which can be further classified as: (1) *vocal qualities*: volume, rhythm, pitch and inflection (modification of vocal units in phoneme articulation) and (2) *vocalizations*: vocal characterizers (crying, laugh, etc.), vocal qualifiers (similar to vocal qualities but modifying only small segment of the sentence in order, for instance, to stress particular elements), and vocal segregates (short, non-lexical elements, e.g., mhm, shhh). Paralinguistic components are vocal effects perceived as having an intonation, volume, and length in time and are produced and shaped by physiological mechanisms (larynx and the nasal, and oral cavities).

Generally, prosody is considered to be a pivotal element in characterizing the speaker's meaning, as it provides fundamental cues allowing the correct interpretation of sentences [89]. The use of those components requires abilities to decode/encode meanings through non-linguistic indexes. For instance, upon encountering a semantically ambiguous sentence, individuals usually rely on prosodic elements to correctly interpret the speaker's meaning. Moreover, word and sentence meanings can change as a function of the prosodic profile of the utterance: stress distribution and intonation can convey different intentions and, therefore, induce different perlocutory effects. Take, for example, the sentence "No way," uttered by a friend in response to another friend's question, "We are going to the beach. Are you coming along?" Modulation of the prosodic profile of the sentence results in the expression of different intentions and epistemic and emotional states. For instance, a plain intonation connotes the sentence as a mere negation and could be simply interpreted as "No, I'm not," whereas an exclamative intonation can completely change the conveyed meaning by shifting the focus on the preceding sentence "We are going to the beach" such that it is interpreted as "Are you *really* going to the beach?". Finally, through the modulation of the prosodic profile, it is also possible to express mental or emotional states; in this case, disapproval of or disgust for the proposal.

Prosody is in fact particularly relevant to connote the *emotional dimension* of messages. Choices about words together with prosodic modulations and non-verbal elements concur in communicating speakers' attitudes, since the suprasegmental profiles express motivational components and contribute to define the referential meaning of a message.

Prosody can be differentiated along different levels based on its functions: *intrinsic prosody* deals with the intonational profile of sentences and allows, for instance, interrogative sentences to be distinguished from affirmative sentences. *Intellective prosody* is connected with illocutionary force and marks peculiar elements of a sentence in order to express specific intentions and cues about the sentence's correct interpretation (e.g., it is possible to derive the ironic meaning of the utterance "That's just great" by decoding the stress on the word "just"). *Emotional prosody* concerns the vocal expression of emotions, which enables us to distinguish an angry *vs* a sad voice.

Empirical evidence suggests that the right hemisphere is particularly involved in emotional prosody, compared to intrinsic or intellective prosody [89]. Furthermore, there seems to be a double dissociation between prosody production and elaboration processes. In subjects with lesions to right frontal areas, speech can be aprosodic or monotonic. However, in those same subjects the ability to decode and recognize prosodic components in an interlocutor's voice is preserved. By contrast, subjects impaired in prosodic meaning recognition but with unaltered prosody production ability have lesions in posterior areas of the right hemisphere [90].

Of particular interest are prosodic functions oriented to the communication of emotions. The voice can express emotions through the modulations of parameters such as rhythm, intonation, and volume. Different emotions present definite prosodic profiles. Generally it is possible to distinguish two patterns of acoustic characteristics: (1) high fundamental frequency (F_0), volume, and rhythm and (2) low F_0, limited modulation of intonations, low volume, and slow rhythm. Analyzing emotions characterized by one or the other pattern, has led to the conclusion that the first pattern corresponds to emotions defined by high arousal (e.g., happiness, anger, fear), while the second distinguishes emotions with low arousal (e.g., sadness, boredom) [86].

1.5.1.2 Neuropsychological Deficits of Prosody

Analyses of deficits and impairments of prosodic functions rely on methodological paradigms in which subjects are asked to produce sentences with a particular affective vocal pattern or a particular inflection. In the examination of comprehension, subjects are required to identify a particular prosodic profile indexing specific emotional states or denoting specific non-literal meanings (e.g., ironic). It is difficult to classify prosodic deficits since an exhaustive model of normal prosodic performance, including acoustic and physiological parameters, is still lacking [86]. The most common disorders of prosodic functions are: (1) *disprosody*, intended as the modification of vocal qualities, generally associated with non-fluent aphasia and lesions to the right hemisphere. In this case, emotional components can remain unaltered, with compromise limited to articulation, pronunciation, and intonation processes; (2) *aprosody*, denoting constriction or lack of prosodic variations in speech, as is common in Parkinson's disease; and (3) *hyperprosody*, involving a disproportionate and accentuated use of prosody, often observed in manic disorders.

Deficits to prosodic function are often consequence of lesions to the right hemisphere. However in some aphasic patients there is a positive correlation between sentence comprehension and prosodic profile decoding, in particular concerning emotional prosody. According to those data, left hemisphere lesions that compromise language comprehension can also compromise prosodic aspects of speech. It must be noted, however, that paralanguage decoding is based on the ability to elaborate phonetic material. Therefore, linguistic disorders involving deficits in the elaboration of phonetic units can result in the compromise of prosody decoding abilities.

Regarding emotional prosody, sub-cortical dysfunctions have been associated with production and comprehension deficits [91]. The basal ganglia seem to be involved in emotional prosody. Moreover, monotonic speech is associated with lesions of the right hemisphere as well as the left hemisphere and sub-cortical structures. Variations in normative values of F_0 have been reported in subjects with lesions to either the right or the left hemisphere [92, 93].

Right hemispheric dominance for emotional components has been explained by different theories. The *perceptive hypothesis* suggests that the right hemisphere is favored in the elaboration of acoustic stimuli; a *functional hypothesis*, on the other hand, assumes that emotional cues without semiotic value are the specific competence of the right hemisphere (see [90] for a review). The left hemisphere, however, is involved in the elaboration of vocal affective components. Right hemispheric dominance is limited to non-verbal affective components, distinct from emotional semantic ones, that is, the ability to label emotions and define their meaning as a function of a specific context. Therefore, both hemispheres participate in the comprehension of affective prosodic components. In fact, deficits in affective prosody decoding have been reported in patients with left hemispheric lesions; at the same time, a bilateral activation was recorded in a prosodic decoding task [94], endorsing hypotheses of a "relative" dominance for the right hemisphere. Recent models suggest that the left hemisphere performs integrative functions, combining outputs of emotional-vocal-related processes and verbal-semantic processes [92].

1.5.2 Indirect Speech Acts and Pragmatic Functions of Figurative Language

The right hemisphere seems to have a specific competence also for pragmatic functions of language, specifically, the use of words in context. The relation between pragmatics and neuropsychology allows two crucial aspects to be addressed: the *cognitive components* in the production/elaboration of non-standard meanings [95] and the *specificity of pragmatic functions*, precisely, the question of their dependence/independence from other levels of linguistic componential structure [24].

Pragmatic functions pertain to all levels of language and communication (see Chapter 5). In this paragraph; we describe two phenomena. In the first, *indirect acts of speech and implicit communication*, the right hemisphere appears to be specifically involved in the elaboration of implicit meanings. Subjects with lesion to the right brain are unable to correctly evaluate contextual meanings and therefore to correctly comprehend the non-explicit components of messages, such as pretences and allusions [96]. Moreover, these patients are impaired in their comprehension of indirect requests. Those deficits show the inability of right-brain-damaged subjects to activate the representational models that are coherent with communicative context [97]. The focus of interest of the second phenomenon, *figurative language,* is the cognitive operations enabling a shift from the direct to the indirect level of encoding/decoding. Different pragmatic models have produced different descriptions as to how figurative and non-figurative meaning is processed and how it is related to different pathways of elaboration (see Chaps. 5 and 6). However, both indirect speech acts and figurative language require skilled inferential abilities in order to be correctly decoded [98]. In fact, the interpretative process oriented to implicit meaning

1

comprehension requires a large amount of prior linguistic and contextual information in order to be successful.

Finally, it is necessary to note the still open question regarding the *functional modularity* of pragmatic functions supporting language production/comprehension, and the implied *structural modularity* of cortical regions involved in pragmatic elaboration. To address this question, it is first necessary to determine whether pragmatic functions are separate from general linguistic and communicative functions, as far as *cognitive processes* and *cortical structures* are concerned. Second, it is necessary to establish whether pragmatic functions are *temporally* distinguished by linguistic functions (see also Chapter 5).

1.6 Discourse Neuropragmatics

A neuropragmatic analysis of discourse focuses on the super-sentential level, examining superordinate processes involved in the production and comprehension of articulated communicative units and an understanding of their structure. In particular, discourse neuropragmatics examines a speaker's compentence in constructing and comprehending speech units, defining logical sequences and focusing on the most relevant elements [99].

Recent empirical evidence has underlined the role of the right hemisphere in discourse production and comprehension, with regard to its abilities to organize sentences and to evaluate their relevance such that the global meaning of the discourse can be understood [100]. Individuals with focal damage to the left hemisphere show difficulties in detecting the thematic elements of stories and in using a story's elements to build a global representation of discourse meaning [101]. Similar results were reported in studies on discourse coherence [39] and discourse intrinsic meaning comprehension [102]. In the latter, PET analysis evidenced major activation of the right inferior frontal gyrus and the right medial temporal gyrus.

1.6.1 Discourse Competences: the Kintsch and van Dijk Model

In general, discourse competence presupposes the ability to activate a multilevel cognitive process aimed at conceptualizing single units as a unique global configuration. This competence involves the integration of several functional levels, requiring, in turn, a global representation of information obtained through specific inferential processes. Empirical studies have focused mostly on lexical and morphosyntactic coherence, using, among others, grammatical and semantic indexes such as type/token ratio (a lexical variability index), indexes related to discourse global structure such as sentences length and number [103], or elements that can be connected to the semantic structure of the discourse [104]. Sometimes, indirect measures of discourse cohesion have been used (anaphors, lexical repetitions, synonymia, etc.) to elucidate the degree of discourse coherence.

The aim of the model proposed by Kintsch and van Dijk [105] was to predict crucial mechanisms in discourse production and comprehension. Its main focus is meta-level units, such as meta-phrasal elements, which are sentence structures organized through rules and relations among sub-units (causal, sequential, etc.). Those units can include episodes, in turn constituted by sub-units, such as setting, characters, aims, and roles. On a cognitive level, all those units and their reciprocal relations should be adequately represented in a macro-structure, especially with respect to causal relations [106]. According to the model, interpreting a text is a complex process, one that requires the on-line integration of information and which is constrained by working memory span limits. Therefore, the analysis and interpretation of textual elements occurs in cyclical phases in which micro-propositions (verb + argument) are hierachically organized within networks and linked together to form a thematic unit, which represents the focal element of discourse structure. Thematic attribution allows indefinite or ambiguous information to be interpreted, facilitates inferences about what has not been explicitly stated, and biases anticipation about subsequent information, by determining a system of semantic expectancies.

On the cognitive side, comprehension may be more or less complex, depending on the cognitive efforts required to connect different parts of discourse into a coherent representation. Thus, comprehension requires inferential processes engaged in an active task of construction/re-construction of a text and the application of adequate contextual heursitics in order to define discourse themes. In this regard, the right hemisphere exhibits a unique competence related to meaning attribution, based on the general organization of thematic components hierarchically ordered, from the analytic (micro-structure) to the global (macro-structure) level. Subjects with lesions to the right hemisphere show deficits in constructing the global gist of discourse, in making inferences about what has been said, and in selecting relevant information [100].

1.7 Conversational Functions

Pragmatic functions for conversation deal mostly with the attunement and adjustment of interactive exchange dynamics. Conversation can be represented as a goal-oriented interaction within spatial-temporal coordinates. It requires specific and complex cognitive and social abilites as well as linguistic and pragmatic skills, which can be included in the general domain of interaction management and behavior adjustment within social contexts.

Neurolinguistics has adopted Gricean pragmatics [22] as a general model of conversation regulation. More recently, some models have focused on the role of conversational implicatures [32, 75] in order to highlight the role of inferential processes regulating mutual interchange. On the cognitive level, the ensemble of representations constitutes *background knowledge*, which frames the interaction and guarantees coherence and relevance to the interactive dynamic: relevant knowledge representations together with mutually shared contextual information form the shared environment that shapes communicative dynamics and processes. Following these approaches, representational elements of conversation are progressively integrated into speakers' mental models, thus increasing the mutual background.

However, for the analysis of conversation adjustment, two elements are fundamental: *local coherence* and *global plausibility*. Coherence, in particular, is based on the regulation of superimpositions, thematic progression, logical coherence, and the pragmatic relevance of discourse [25]. Another crucial element for the analysis of communicative exchanges is the turn-taking rule [107]. Conversational turns are selected and taken, for instance, by elevating one's tone of voice and selecting one's interlocutor through verbal or non-verbal acts. Finally, the types of produced sentences and speech acts are relevant aspect of conversation, since they have a direct impact on interpretative processes.

More specifically, inabilities to modulate turn-taking, speech style or to attune one's communicative register to the wider conversational context are attributed to impaired social communicative competencies. Generally, those deficits are considered as interpersonal communication disorders and include inabilities in contextualizing events and evaluating their plausibility, with consequential inabilities in grasping the global gist of conversational scripts. Finally, the inability to understand and use mutual knowledge has been linked with more general deficits in meta-representational abilities and social cognition (see Chapter 9).

In an attempt to integrate different components involved in conversation production and comprehension, Frederiksen and colleagues [108] proposed a model that refers to the semantic-pragmatic level and to the conceptual components necessary to regulate communicative exchange. The model defines the communicative process as a sequence of natural language expressions that encode only part of the wider conceptual knowledge possessed by the speaker. It operates simultaneously on four different levels: *linguistic*, *propositional*, *semantic-pragmatic*, and *conceptual*. The conceptual component, in particular, is a mental representation (or model) of information, originating partly from long-term memory and partly from discourse context. The latter, in turn, develops following an incremental process that unfolds as the conversation advances and it frames the interpretation of discourse units. The four levels represent functionally distinct processes. Empirical data regarding focal deficits in specific functions support the existence of autonomous modules: in some cases, a preserved competence in local interpretation is followed by pragmatic deficits. Subjects with damage to language areas of the left hemisphere show impairments in the indirect elaboration of requests or in figurative language comprehension.

References

1. Brown CM, Hagoort P (1999) The neurocognition of language: challenges and future directions. In: Brown CM, Hagoort P (Eds) The neurocognition of language. Oxford University Press, New York, pp 3-15

2. Jackendoff R (1999) The representational structure of the language faculty and their interactions. In: Brown CM, Hagoort P (eds) The neurocognition of language. Oxford University Press, New York, pp 37-79
3. Stemmer B, Whitaker HA (1998) Handbook of neurolinguistics. Academic, San Diego
4. Seidemberg MS (1995) Visual recognition: an overview. In: Miller JL, Eimas PD (eds) Speech, language and communication. Academic, New York, pp 138-179
5. Deacon TW (1997) The symbolic Species: the co-evolution of language and the brain. Norton, New York
6. Rugg MD (1999) Functional neuroimaging in cognitive neuroscience. In: Brown CM, Hagoort P (eds) The neurocognition of language. Oxford University Press, New York, pp 37-79
7. Frazier L (1995) Issues of representation in psycholinguistics. In: Miller JL, Eimas PD (eds) Speech, language and communication. Academic Press, New York, pp 1-29
8. Levelt WJM (1999) Producing spoken language: a blueprint of the speaker. In: Brown CM, Hagoort P (eds) The neurocognition of language. Oxford University Press, New York, pp 83-122
9. Caramazza A (2000) The organization of conceptual knowledge in the brain. In: Gazzaniga M (ed) The new cognitive neuroscience. Bradford Book/The MIT Press, Cambridge Mass, pp 1037-1046
10. Miceli G, Caramazza A (1988) Dissociation of inflectional and derivational morphology. Brain Lang 35:24-65
11. Zaidel E (1990) Language functions in the two hemispheres following cerebral commissurotomy and hemispherectomy. In: Boller F, Grafman J (eds) Handbook of neuropsychology. Elsevier, Amsterdam, pp 115-150
12. Noveck IA, Sperber D (2004) Experimental pragmatics. Palgrave, San Diego
13. Van Berkum JJA (in press) The electrophysiology of discourse and conversation. In: Spivey M, Joanisse M, McRae K (eds) The Cambridge handbook of psycholinguistics. Cambridge University Press, New York
14. Basso A, Cubelli R (1999) Clinical aspects of aphasia. In: Pizzamiglio L, Denes G (eds) Handbook of clinical neuropsychology. Psychology Press, Hove, pp 181-193
15. Damasio AR, Damasio H (2000) Aphasia and the neural basis of language. In: Mesulam MM (ed) Principles of behavioral and cognitive neurology. Oxford University Press, New York, pp 294-315
16. Làdavas E, Berti AE (2009) Neuropsicologia [Neuropsychology]. Il Mulino, Bologna
17. Carston R (2002) Linguistic meaning, communicated meaning and cognitive pragmatics. Mind Lang 17:127-148
18. Kasher A (1994) Modular speech act theory: programme and results. In: Tsohatzidis SL (ed) Foundations of speech act theory. Routledge, London, pp 312-322
19. Büchel C, Frith C, Friston K (1999) Functional integration: methods for assessing interactions among neuronal systems using brain imaging. In: Brown CM, Hagoort P (eds) The neurocognition of language. Oxford University Press, New York, pp 337-358
20. Katrin A (2009) Architectonic language research. In: Stemmer B, Whitaker HA (eds) Handbook of the neuroscience of language. Elsevier, Amsterdam, pp 33-44
21. Demonet JF (1998) Tomographic brain imaging of language functions: prospects for a new brain/language model. In: Stemmer B, Whitaker HA (eds) Handbook of neurolinguistics. Academic, San Diego, pp 132-143
22. Grice HP (1989) Studies in the way of words. Harvard University Press, Cambridge
23. Searle JR (1979) Expression and meaning. Cambridge University Press, Cambridge
24. Bar-Hillel Y (1971) Pragmatics of natural language. Reidel, Dordrecht
25. Sperber D, Wilson D (1986) Relevance: communication and cognition. Oxford University Press, Oxford
26. Baron-Cohen S (1995) Mindblindness: an essay on autism and theory of mind. The MIT Press, Cambridge

27. Frith CD, Wolpert DM (2004) The neuroscience of social interaction: decoding, imitating and influencing the actions of others. Oxford University Press, Oxford
28. Mitchell JP, Mason MF, Macrae CN, Banaji MR (2006) Thinking about others: the neural substrates of social cognition. In: Cacioppo JT, Visser PS, Pickett CL (eds) Social neuroscience: people thinking about thinking people. The MIT Press, Cambridge, pp 63-82
29. Sally D (2004) Dressing the mind properly for the game. In: Frith CD, Wolpert DM (eds) The neuroscience of social interaction: decoding, imitating and influencing the actions of others. Oxford University Press, Oxford, pp 283-303
30. Gallese V (2001) The "shared manifold" hypothesis: from mirror neurons to empathy. J Consc Stud 8:33-50
31. Bara B, Tirassa M (2000) Neuropragmatics: brain and communication. Brain Lang 71:10-14
32. Lakoff G, Johnson M (1980) Metaphors we live by. University of Chicago Press, Chicago
33. Shank R, Abelson R (1977) Scripts, plans, goals and understanding. Erlbaum, Hillsdale, New Jersey
34. Cacioppo JT, Visser PS, Pickett CL (2006) Social neuroscience: people thinking about thinking people. The MIT Press, Cambridge, Mass
35. Lorch MP, Borod JC, Koff E (1998) The role of emotion in the linguistic and pragmatic aspects of aphasic performance. J Neuroling 11:103-118
36. Giora R (2003) On our mind: Salience, context and figurative language. Oxford University Press, New York
37. Giora R (1999) On the priority of salient meanings: studies of literal and figurative language. J Pragmatics 31:919-929
38. Stemmer B, Giroux F, Joanette Y (1994) Production and evaluation of requests by right hemisphere brain-damaged individuals. Brain Lang 47:1-31
39. Maguire EA, Frith CD, Morris RGR (1999) The functional neuroanatomy of comprehension and memory: the importance of prior knowledge. Brain 122:1839- 1850
40. Robertson DA, Gernsbacher MA, Guidotti SJ et al (2000) Functional neuroanatomy of the cognitive process of mapping during discourse comprehension. Psychol Sci 11:255-260
41. Balconi M, Carrera A (2006) Cross-modal perception of emotional face and voice. A neuropsychological approach. Paper presented at the "2th Meeting of the European Societies of Neuropsychology" (18-20 October), Toulouse, France
42. Calvert GA, Campbell R, Brammer MJ (2000) Evidence from functional magnetic resonance imaging of crossmodal binding in the human heteromodal cortex. Curr Biol 10:649-657
43. Giles H, Smith P (1979) Accommodation theory: optimal levels of convergence. In: Giles H, St. Clair H (eds) Language and social psychology. Basil Blackwell, Oxford
44. Pickering MJ, Garrod S (2003) Toward a mechanistic psychology of dialogue. Behav Brain Sci 26:678-678
45. Hickock G (2000) Speech perception, conduction aphasia and the functional neuroatonomy of language. In: Grodzinsky Y, Shapiro LP, Swinney D (eds) Language and the brain: representation and processes. Academic, San Diego, pp 87-104
46. Hiscock M (1998) Brain lateralization across life span. In: Stemmer B, Whitaker HA (eds) Handbook of neurolinguistics. Academic, San Diego, pp 358-368
47. Zaidel E (1998) Language in the right emisphere following callosal disconnection. In: Stemmer B, Whitaker HA (eds) Handbook of neurolinguistics. Academic, San Diego, pp 369-383
48. Banich MT (1997) Neuropsychology: the neural bases of mental function. Houghton Mifflin, Boston
49. Hellige JB (1998) Unity of language and communication: interhemispheric interaction in the lateralized brain. In: Stemmer B, Whitaker HA (eds) Handbook of neurolinguistics. Academic, San Diego, pp 405-414
50. Lieberman P (2000) Human language and the reptilian brain. Harvard University Press, Cambridge Mass

51. Crosson B, Nadeau SE (1998) The role of subcortical structures in linguistic processes: recent developments. In: Stemmer B, Whitaker HA (eds) Handbook of neurolinguistics. Academic, San Diego, pp 431-445
52. Damasio AR, Damasio H (1992) Brain and language. Sci Am 267:88-95
53. Creutzfeldt O, Ojemann, G, Lettich E (1989) Neuronal activity in the human lateral temporal lobe: I. Responses to speech. Exp Brain Res 77:451-475
54. Boatman D, Hart JJ, Lesser RP et al (1998) Right hemisphere speech perception revealed by amobarbital injection and electrical interference. Neurology 51:458-464
55. Zaidel E (1985) Language in the right hemisphere. In: Benson DF, zaidel E (eds) The dual brain: hemispheric specialisation in humans. Guilford, New York, pp 205-231
56. Levelt WJM, Praamastra P, Meyer AS et al (1998) An MEG study of picture naming. J Cognitive Neurosci 10:553-567
57. Warren RM (1968) Verbal transformation effect and auditory perceptual mechanisms. Psychological Bulletin 70:261-270
58. Damasio AR (1989) The brain binds entities and events by multiregional activation from convergence zones. Neural Comput 1:123-132
59. Mesulam MM (1998) From sensation to cognition. Brain 121:1013-1052
60. Garret MF (1992) Disorders of lexical selection. Cognition 42:143-180
61. Levelt WJM (1989) Speaking: from intention to articulation. The MIT Press, Cambridge Mass
62. Vigliocco G, Antonini T, Garret MF (1998) Grammatical gender is on the tip of Italian tongues. Psychol Sci 8:314-317
63. McCarthy R, Warrington EK (1984) A two-route model of speech production. Evidence from aphasia. Brain 107:463-485
64. Damasio H, Grabowsky TJ, Tranel D et al (1996) A neural basis for lexical retrieval. Nature 380:499-505
65. Miceli G, Silveri MC, Nocentini U, Caramazza A (1988) Patterns of dissociationin comprehension and production of nouns and verbs. Aphasiology 2:351-358
66. Garret M (2000) Remarks on the architecture of language processing systems. In: Grodzinsky Y, Shapiro LP, Swinney D (eds) Language and the brain: representation and processes. Academic, San Diego, pp 31-69
67. Hagoort P, Brown CM, Osterhout L (1999) The neurocognition of syntactic processing. In: Brown CM, Hagoort P (eds) The neurocognition of language. Oxford University Press, New York, pp 273-315
68. Frazier L (1987) Processing syntactic structures: evidence from Dutch. Nat Lang Linguist Th 5:519-559
69. Frazier L (1990) Exploring the architecture of language processing system. In: Altmann MT (ed) Cognitive model of speech processing: psycholinguistic and computational processing. The MIT Press, Cambridge, Mass, pp 409-433
70. Kutas M, Hillyard S (1984) Brain potential during reading reflects word expectancies and semantic association. Nature 307:161-163
71. Federmeier KD, Kutas M (2003) Il linguaggio del cervello [The brain language]. In: Zani A, Mado Proverbio A (eds) Elettrofisiologia della mente [Electrophysiology of mind]. Carocci, Roma, pp 139-171
72. Balconi M, Pozzoli U (2004) Elaborazione di anomalie semantiche e sintattiche con stimolazione visiva e uditiva. Un'analisi mediante correlati ERPs [Semantic and syntactic anomalies processing with visual and auditory stimulation. An analysis through ERP correlates]. GIP 3:585-612
73. Beeman M, Chiarello C (1998) Right hemisphere language comprehension: perspectives from cognitive neuroscience. Erlbaum, Hillsdale

1

74. Lakoff G (1987) Women, fire and dangerous things: what categories reveal about the mind. University of Chicago Press, Chicago
75. Levinson SC (2000) Presumptive meanings: the theory of generalized conversational implicature. The MIT Press, Cambridge, Mass
76. Mininni G (2000) Psicologia del parlare comune [Psychology of common speaking]. Editoriale Grasso, Bologna
77. Messing LS, Campbell R (1999) Gesture, speech and sign. Oxford University Press, Oxford
78. Dennet DC (1987) The intentional stance. The MIT Press, Cambridge
79. Searle JR (1983) Intentionality: an essay in the philosophy of mind. Cambridge University Press, Cambridge
80. Gardner H, Brownell HH (1986) Right hemisphere communication battery. Psychology Service, Boston
81. Nusbaum HC, Small SL (2006) Investigating cortical mechanisms of language processing in social context. In: Cacioppo JT, Visser PS, Pickett CL (eds) Social neuroscience: people thinking about thinking people. The MIT Press, Cambridge, pp 131-152
82. Puce A, Perret D (2004) Electrophisiology and brain imaging of biological motion. In: Frith CD, Wolpert DM (eds) The neuroscience of social interaction: decoding, imitating and influencing the actions of others. Oxford University Press, New York, pp 1-22
83. Campell R, MacSweeney M, Surguladze S et al (2001) Cortical substrates for the perception of face actions: an fMRI study of the specificità of activation for seen speech and for meaningless lower-face acts (gurning). Cognitive Brain Res 12:233-243
84. Rizzolatti G, Craighero L, Fadiga L (2002) The mirror system in humans. In: Stamenov MI, Gallese V (eds) Mirror neurons and the evolution of brain and language. John Benjamins, Amsterdam, pp 37–59
85. Goldin-Meadow S, Nusbaum H, Kelly SD, Wagner S (2001) Explaining math: gesturing lightens the load. Psychol Sci 12:516-522
86. Davidson RJ, Scherer KR, Hill Goldsmith H (2003) Handbook of affective sciences. Oxford University Press, New York
87. Siegman AW, Feldstein S (1987) Nonverbal behavior and communication. Erlbaum, Hillsdale
88. Trager GL (1958) Paralanguage: a first approximation. Stud Linguist 13:1-12
89. Ross ED (2000) Affective prosody and the aprosodias. In: Mesulam MM (ed) Principles of behavioral and cognitive neurology. Oxford University Press, New York, pp 316-331
90. Pell MD (2006) Cerebral mechanisms for understanding emotional prosody in speech. Brain Lang 96:221-234
91. Denes G, Caldognetto EM, Semenza C et al (1984) Discriminationand identification of emotions in human voice by brain damaged subjects. Acta Neurol Scand 69:154-162
92. Friederici AD, Alter K (2004) Lateralization of auditory language functions: a dynamic dual pathway model. Brain Lang 89:267-276
93. Kotz S, Meyer M, Alter K et al (2003) On the lateralization of emotional prosody: An event-related functional MR investigation. Brain Lang 86:366-376
94. Gandour J, Tong Y, Wong D et al (2004) Hemispheric roles in the perception of speech prosody. Neuroimage 23:344-357
95. Marraffa M (2005) Meccanismi della comunicazione. In: Ferretti F, Gambarara D (eds) Comunicazione e scienza cognitive. Laterza, Roma, pp 151
96. Anolli L, Balconi M, Ciceri R (2002) Deceptive miscommunication theory (DeMiT): a new model for the analysis of deceptive communication. In: Anolli L, Ciceri R, Riva G (eds) Say not to say: new perspectives on miscommunication. Ios Press, Amsterdam, pp 75-104
97. Beeman M (1998) Coarse semantic coding and discourse comprehension. In: Beeman M, Chiarello C (eds) Right hemisphere language comprehension: perspectives from cognitive neuroscience. Erlbaum, Hillsdale, pp 255-284

98. Verschueren J (1999) Understanding pragmatics. Arnold, London
99. Kintsch W (1998) Comprehension: a paradigm for cognition. Cambridge University Press, Cambridge
100. Rehak A, Kaplan JA, Weylman ST et al (1992) Story processing in right brain damaged patients. Brain Lang 42:320-336
101. Caplan R, Dapretto M (2001) Making sense during conversation. NeuroReport 12:3625-3632
102. Nichelli P, Grafman J, Pietrini P et al (1995) Where the brain appreciates the moral of a story. Neuroreport 6:2309-2313
103. Ulatowska HK, North AJ, Macaluso-Haynes S (1981) Production of narrative and procedural discourse in aphasia. Brain Lang 13:345-371
104. Chapman SB, Ulatowska HA (1989) Discourse in aphasia: Integration deficits in processing reference. Brain Lang 36:651-668
105. van Dijk TA, Kintsch W (1983) Strategies of discourse comprehension. Academic Press, New York
106. Kintsch W, van Dijk TA (1978) Toward a model of text comprehension and production. Psychol Rev 85:363-394
107. Schegloff EA (1972) Sequencing in conversational openings. In: Gumperz JJ, Hymes DH (eds) Directions in sociolinguistics. Holt, New York, pp 346-380
108. Frederiksen CH, Bracewell RJ, Breuleux A, Renaud A (1990) The cognitive representation and processing of discourse: function and dysfunction. In: Joanette Y, Brownell H (eds) Discourse ability and brain damage: theoretical and empirical perspectives. Springer, New York, pp 19-44

Methods and Research Perspectives on the Neuropsychology of Communication

2

M. Balconi

2.1 Introduction

The introduction of advanced instruments and methodologies of analysis has led to important scientific contributions in the study of communicative and linguistic processes, allowing researchers to explore at deeper levels the functional architecture of brain structures underlying language and communication [1]. This chapter provides an introduction to the methodologies used in the study of language and communication. In particular, we discuss the advances introduced by the neuropsychological paradigm–on both the experimental and the clinical level–regarding the exploration of basic functions of communicative processes. In addition, we describe the broad panorama comprising the major psychophysiological (e.g., the analysis of event-related potentials, ERPs) and neuropsychological instruments (e.g., neuroimaging techniques) used to better define the contribution of cortical areas to communication. For each methodology and paradigm introduced, the most important empirical contributions and critical issues are discussed.

2.2 Assumptions of Cognitive Neuropsychology

2.2.1 Function-structure Relationship

The basic assumption of the neuropsychological approach is the existence of a relation between *anatomico-structural components* and *cognitive functions* [2, 3]. Two

M. Balconi (✉)
Department of Psychology, Catholic University of Milan, Milan, Italy

issues are central to this assumption: there is a direct link between functional units and brain structures, and the representation of brain structure is qualitatively invariant, notwithstanding lesions and damage [1]. In other words, as cognitive neuropsychology studies have considered especially those patients with brain focal lesions in order to make inferences regarding the normal functioning of a cognitive system, it has become necessary to elucidate the correspondence between the brain's neural structure and its functional organization. If process-distinguished mental operations are founded on partially separated physical processes (brain structures), then a focal lesion may selectively damage one function without affecting the others.

The analysis of anatomic-structural correlates of communicative functions should consider two fundamental aspects: (a) the dichotomy between *localism* (which hypothesizes a one-to-one correspondence between specific functions and circumscribed brain areas) and *holism* (which hypothesizes the distribution of communicative functions onto extended brain areas/networks); (b) the issue of *left lateralization* for linguistic competence and the role of the *right hemisphere* in the production and comprehension of messages [4].

In the classical models of neuropsychology, the relation between brain anatomy and cognitive functions demand an exact collocation of cognitive functions within circumscribed brain areas. By contrast, anti-localist models reject a modular approach and instead favor a correspondence between function and underlying anatomic structure via complex networks and involving several brain areas [5].

Modern cognitive neuropsychology views the correspondence between cognitive modules and neural structures in terms of brain networks, thus involving a plurality of brain regions. These models accept the *polyfunctionality* of brain areas, according to which the same neural circuit can be implicated in a plurality of cognitive functions, thus operating in several cognitive processes but potentially in different roles. The localist view may be applicable to simple communicative functions (e.g., phonological representation of linguistic inputs) but it is more difficult to single out circumscribed localizations for complex functions, such as discourse planning, control and monitoring, or verbal and non-verbal integration.

2.2.2
Structural, Functional and Representational Modularity

In this paragraph we introduce the concept of "module" (and thus of "modularity"), considering the evolution of the respective ideas over the last few decades. During that time, different approaches to modularity have produced different theoretical views, ranging from a strict version, which assumes the existence of local, anatomically distinguished and functionally independent sub-systems [6], to more moderate versions, which refer to a more complex architecture involved in cognitive functions [7]. Nonetheless, views of modularity have commonly hypothesized a correspondence between neural structure and the mind's functional organization. This view is endorsed by experimental findings related to correlations between lesions of specific areas and deficits of defined cognitive functions (see also Par. 2.3). However, as already mentioned, although in some cases it is possible to draw a strong correlation between cognitive functions and specific cerebral areas, precise localization is more difficult for complex, higher cognitive processes.

Recently, the concept of modularity has been further developed, with *representational modularity* [8] replacing previous acceptance of functional modularity. Accordingly, modularity no longer refers to general processes such as language perception, but to integrative and inferential processes. In other words, the domain specificity of mental processes is based on the representations to which they have access or derive from. It is thus a definition of modularity that deals with integrative processes (e.g., syntactic parsing operates on sequences of lexical categories in order to construct correct syntactic structures) and inferential operations (e.g., processes operating to translate a representational format into another format).

2.3 Methods of Analysis in Cognitive Neuropsychology

2.3.1 Experimental and Clinical Methods

Early studies of the cognitive functions involved in language and communication were conducted on single cases and thus described circumscribed and localized deficits, such as in word reading or sentence comprehension. One of the principal advantages provided by clinical methodology is the possibility to prove the independence of cognitive operation through the existence of *functional dissociations* and *double dissociations* (see previous paragraph, [1]). In addition, the analysis of single unit dysfunctions may suggest the functioning of the same unit under normal conditions. In other words, empirical evidence on brain-damaged subjects has allowed inferences to be made regarding the functional organization of processes operative in healthy conditions. However, only recently has it been possible to directly analyze cognitive functioning in healthy subjects, using advanced technologies and improved experimental methodologies [9].

In light of the evolution of neuropsychology as a discipline, we introduce the distinction between *experimental* and *clinical* methodologies. A common assumption underlying both approaches is the cognitive model, which aims to dissect the entire communicative process as a virtual sequence of process-based phases, in which information, in different representational formats, flows from one process-based component to another, during which it undergoes specific transformations [10]. It is necessary to note that cognitive neuropsychology aims to dissect cognitive functions into their basic components [3]. In experimental neuropsychology, the analysis involves healthy subjects and the study of processes underlying communicative competence (e.g., the comprehension of anaphors).

Besides the instruments used, the two methods can be differentiated on the basis of the *samples*. In some cases, the studies involve a single subject, while, in other cases the analysis draws on groups of subjects with deficits in the same cognitive operation [11]. Let us compare the two methodologies: in *single-case studies*, a specific disorder in a certain cognitive function (e.g., the comprehension of emotional prosody) may be caused by a circumscribed brain lesion, detectable through the analysis of single clinical cases. This perspective has resulted in localist models of cerebral functions. In *group studies*, by contrast, comparisons are made between healthy and brain-damaged subjects thorough quantitative methods (usually tests). Moreover, group studies, unlike single-case studies, permit a reliable statistical analysis, thus overcoming the limits imposed on classical neuropsychological studies. The primary aim of these studies is to define specific levels of deficit in certain communicative modalities. With the recent developments in psychodiagnostics, those studies now include controlled evaluation procedures and standardized psychometric tools that allow the selection of homogeneous subject cohorts. But how are groups created? Both the homogeneity of the subjects' symptomatology and the site of their cerebral lesions must be considered. Therefore, the analysis examines the presence/absence of certain symptomatologies when lesions to specific brain areas occur.

2.4 Neuropsychological Measures for Language and Communication

Putting aside the potential methodological implications deriving from the use of different measuring tools, we now review the main indexes for the study of communication, paying particular attention to psychophysiological and neuropsychological measures.

2.4.1 Neuropsychological Assessment and Psychometric Batteries

The evaluation of linguistic and communicative competencies allows the definition of general working level of specific functions, such as phono-articulatory, grammatical, morphological, syntactic, semantic, and pragmatic properties [1] (for a definition of these levels, see Chapter 1). *Neuropsychological assessment* is the most frequently used procedure within the clinical field [12]. It allows evaluation of the existence and pervasiveness of specific deficits, and, on a behavioral level, the qualitative assessment of both patient performance and the compensatory strategies adopted to cope with impairments arising from damaged functions [13]. Assessment generally includes a broad-spectrum screening, followed by a more detailed evaluation of the damaged functions. This last phase is part of a more articulated procedure that includes case history, clinical interview, clinical evaluation, and indications for rehabilitative intervention.

Psychometric tools (tests), used for the evaluation of communicative competence, generally permit the isolated analysis of certain functional components such as morphosyntactic, lexical, phonological, or semantic abilities [13, 14]. By separating the measurement of linguistic abilities from that of communicative abilities, it is possible to determine that the linguistic results are richer than those reflecting communication/pragmatics. Furthermore, it is possible to divide linguistic tests into different sub-categories: *screening*, *global linguistic functioning*, and *specific linguistic abilities* (see [15] for a review). Of particular interest is the *category of verbal fluency tests* (e.g. [16]). Examples of interesting applications of psychometric indexes have been provided by Hillis and Caramazza [17], in a detailed comparison between deficit typologies. That study allowed the subsequent modeling of language functioning with respect to specific functions. It also yielded an excellent analytic description of deficits as well as good ecological validity, thus demonstrating the highly heuristic value of psychometric indexes, especially in terms of the possibility to define which component of the system is damaged as a result of a particular lesion. However, these studies are less effective in their description of *how* the linguistic system is impaired when certain mechanisms are defective.

More recently, it has been possible to employ instruments more relevant to the areas of the brain involved in higher communicative functions, with the aim of investigating a broader range of competencies in impaired conditions (for a review, see [14]). First, it is possible to distinguish between *pragmatic protocols* and *communicative efficiency tests* [18]. The former aim to evaluate pragmatic aspects of language; for example, the *pragmatic protocol* described in [19] investigates, through 30 behavioral categories, the subject's communication modalities (fluency, prosody, non-verbal components), communicative style, and intentional level (intention formulation and feedback monitoring). The *Profile of Communicative Appropriateness* (PCA) [20] involves a face-to-face interview between subject and experimenter, who, in turn, evaluates the subject's spontaneous speech production through a coding process based on textual models. Specifically, the PCA analyzes responsiveness to the interlocutor's verbal prompts, control of semantic content, cohesion of discourse informative units, verbal fluency, sensitivity to social and relational context, and non-verbal communication. Other protocols are: the *Porch Index of Communicative Abilities* (PICA, [21, 22]), which is used to quantify, among other things, language production and comprehension, reading and writing competence, gesture analysis; the *Communicative Abilities in Daily Living* (CADL, [23]), which estimates a subject's ability to communicate in daily situations; and finally, the *Discourse Comprehension Test* [24], which is one of the most interesting protocols dealing with conversational and discourse elements, as it investigates an individual's ability to understand macro-units of content (see also Chapter 1).

2.4.2 Observational Indexes

One of the main advantages of observational methods is that information about linguistic and communicative functioning can be obtained during the process. Here we consider observational indexes of verbal and non-verbal communication, which are used to analyze mimic and gestural behavior, vocal components, and cognitive indexes, such as response time (RT) and eye movements.

2.4.2.1
Non-verbal Indexes and Response Times

Non-verbal communication is often studied through the use of observational grids for different communicative systems. In fact, it is possible to code a number of signals representative of different communicative channels, including mimic and postural components, gestural system, space management (proxemics), and vocal components.

In a study by Ekman [25], a tool was designed to analyze emotions through facial expressions. The *Facial Action Coding System* (FACS) is aimed at distinguishing basic facial muscular units and defining their role in a global emotional mimic configuration. Indexes such as FACS have been successfully integrated with psychophysiological indexes, such as evoked ERPs (see Par. 2.4.3), in order to more thoroughly study the expression of emotions.

The RT, by contrast, is a chronemic index that is used especially in relation to linguistic tasks. It provides a precise measurement of the time subjects need in order to produce answers related to specific experimental tasks. Although indirect, RT is a more sensitive measure than other behavioral indexes, as differences in RT relative to specific aspects of communication may be detected also in the absence of differences in psychometric scores. RT recording comprises two phases, which permit the dissection of answering processes according to: (a) a *central phase*, in which sensorial information is coded relative to a specific stimulus and an appropriate possible response is selected, and (b) a *peripheral phase*, in which the appropriate motor response is executed (e.g., pressing a key on a keyboard).

In general, RT variations are used as an indirect measure of a task's difficulty, based on the assumption that the more demanding the task (in terms of cognitive effort required for its elaboration), the longer the time needed to perform it. RT has been applied to the study of communicative processes in which the performances of healthy and impaired subjects were compared. For instance, RTs have been used to examine the answers provided by subjects during sentence reading or comprehension tasks, with a focus on semantic processes, as well as to evaluate subjective responses to tasks including semantic ambiguities and polysemy. Finally, on a pragmatic level, RT has been used to investigate abilities in discriminating supra-segmental components.

In recent studies conducted on children, the development of verbal fluency and the strategies used to comprehend sentences were investigated [26]. Both components seem to undergo progressive improvement, as a function of the meta-cognitive strategies that the children developed to produce and comprehend verbal material. In clinical subjects, reported differences in RT have been used to describe the existence of a specific deficit relative to certain operations, such as lexical decision [27] or syntactic elaboration [28], and to evaluate information processing in children with reading impairments [29].

2.4.2.2
Discriminative, Interference and Priming Indexes

A specific category of measures is represented by *discriminative indexes*, which provide useful information for detecting possible differences in the time-course or execution modalities of a single task in the absence of an explicit answer from the subject. Generally, subjects are asked to discriminate between stimuli that differ from each other in terms of temporal boundaries, thus allowing the evaluation of slight differences between processes. For instance, a subject may be asked to discriminate between two ambiguous linguistic stimuli, thus allowing differences in the time-course of processes to be distinguished, as well as testing of the quality of activated representations and the existence of possible associative semantic networks between meanings. Examples of discriminative indexes were provided by Caplan [30], who applied these measures to investigate phoneme confusion in aphasic patients, and by Arguin and colleagues [31], who analyzed the relation between stimuli complexity and semantic organization in category-specific anomy for fruits and vegetables.

Other measures belonging to the same category are represented by *priming* and *interference indexes*. Priming is usually used to facilitate (positive priming) or inhibit (negative priming) access to a second stimulus (target), associated with the first (prime) on a lexical, syntactic, or semantic level. The level of facilitation or interference exerted by priming (measured through RT time-locked to the target) is a measure of the strength and nature of the link between primes and targets, as shown, for instance, in the difficulties in lexical-semantic access observed in patients with Alzheimer's disease [32].

2.4.2.3
Eye Movements

On the behavioral level, measuring eye movements permits evaluation of the cognitive processes underlying the comprehension of written texts [33, 34]. Generally, such movements are monitored through recording tools (such as cameras) equipped with scanning functions. In particular, the electro-oculogram (EOG) measures horizontal and vertical eye movements. The alternation of rapid (a few milliseconds) fixations with saccades (rapid eye shifts) is evidence of text comprehension. Saccadic movements are, in fact, considered an index of meaning elaboration and they are measured in terms of latency, amplitude and direction of movement, etc.

Eye movements are controlled by cortical and sub-cortical systems in conjunction with cranial nerves and ocular muscles. In particular, both the frontal cortex and the occipital cortex are involved in ocular activities: fixations are controlled by the premotor cortex in the frontal lobes, while saccades are regulated by the superior colliculus [35]. Previous studies reported a direct relation between eye movements and cognitive activity, modulated by task complexity. Continuous re-fixations may indicate a subject's need to re-read more ambiguous and/or more complex text elements, thus providing indirect measure of a general comprehension difficulty [36].

Therefore, eye movements are applied to investigate linguistic processes (word or sentence reading) as well as text comprehension. They are directly associated with other phenomena of interest in communication psychology, such as the relationship of *blinking* to the *startle response*, interpreted as a rapid and automatic response to unpredicted stimuli. Increased blinking activity signals the occurrence of an unexpected stimulation. It has been reported that attentive and emotional processes may modulate the startle response, and in general, that a direct relation exists between arousal variations and increasing/decreasing frequencies of blinking [37].

2.4.3 Psychophysiological Indexes: Neurovegetative Measures

Every living organism produces a complex system of physiological "signals" that are connected to its functioning: such units of information are called *biosignals* [37]. It is possible to distinguish two main categories of biosignals on the basis of their nature: *electrical signals*, in the form of biopotentials, are measured by electrocardiogram (ECG), electroencephalogram (EEG), and electromyogram (EMG), while *non-electrical signals* are related to pressure, volumetric, and thermal modifications, among others.

The primary fields of electrophysiological activity are: *skin electrical activity*, which is associated with activation of the neurovegetative system; *eye electrical activity*, comprising *electrical retinal activity* and *eye movements*; and *cerebral activity*, measured as *variations in potentials* and recorded at the scalp level. Autonomic nervous system activation is particularly interesting with respect to non-verbal components of communication [38], especially in relation to the regulation of emotional responses within communicative interactions.

2.4.3.1 Skin Conductance Activity

Skin electrical activity derives from the sympathetic nervous system and is used as an index of subjective emotional activation or reaction level. It is also considered to be a psychogalvanic reflex, or as skin phasic activity, as opposed to tonic activity [39]. The measurement of skin electrical activity involves the recording of spontaneous variations in electric potential between two electrodes placed on the skin (*endogenous*) or of the electrical resistance of the skin produced by the passage of a small amount of current through electrodes (*exogenous* or *skin conductance*). Electrodes are generally positioned on the finger tips, palm of the hand, or on the arm.

Electrodermal activity (EDA) is related to vigilance and orienting processes and has been particularly studied in relation to the communication of emotions, since it indexes emotional unconscious responses in the absence of conscious elaboration of the stimuli. Different studies investigating brain lateralization of emotional responses have shown a major role for the right hemisphere [40, 41]. This hypothesis was confirmed in studies that noted the absence of an EDA response to emotional stimuli (words with emotional values) in right-brain-damaged patients. The right hemisphere therefore appears to be decisive in emotional response production and communication. Studies focusing on the non-verbal communication of emotions evidenced a direct relation between emotional response manipulation and conductance levels. In particular, subjects were asked to increase or decrease their emotional reaction to emotional stimuli [42]; conductance increased when subjects accentuated their reaction and decreased when they diminished their reaction. Non-verbal emotional regulation may thus be supported by specific psychophysiological modifications.

2.4.4 Cortical Electrical Activity

Particular emphasis has been placed on the study of EEG methods, since cortical activity has been extensively assessed in the study of language production and comprehension (see also Chapter 3) and, more recently, in the study of pragmatic components.

2.4.4.1 Electroencephalography

In the EEG, cortical electrical activity is recorded through electrodes placed on the scalp and referred to a common site. Electroencephalographic variations produced by cortical activity can be distinguished in two different indexes: EEG and ERPs. The former is largely employed to investigate neurons synchronous activity compared to basal activity [43]. EEG recording is graphically represented as a continuous sequence of waves with variable frequencies (Fig. 2.1). The rhythmic activity of the

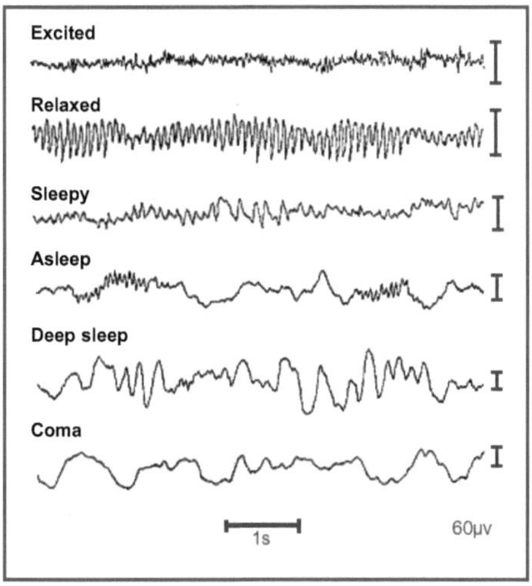

Fig. 2.1 EEG recordings related to the different states of the study subject

2

EEG is divided into five major bands based on frequency. High-voltage (50 μv) and medium-frequency (10 cycles/s) waves are designated as α waves and are typical of the relaxed condition with closed eyes. Waves with low voltage and increased frequency (12–30 Hz) are called β waves. The transition between a resting condition, with the eyes closed, to an alert condition elicits rhythm desynchronization, with subsequent replacement of α waves by β waves. Delta waves (δ) are characterized by their slow frequency (less than 4 Hz) and higher voltage (100 μv) and are typically recorded during deep sleep, while an θ rhythm has a frequency ranging between 4 and 8 Hz and is of high voltage (100 μv). The EEG procedure involves spectrum analysis, the aim of which is to detect the proportion of general electrical activity attributable to each frequency band.

2.4.4.2
Exogenous and Endogenous Event-Related Potentials

The analysis of ERPs consists of the investigation of neural activity linked to repeated external stimuli [44]. ERPs can be defined as the neural response (synaptic response of pyramidal cells dendrites) to brief stimulations. For this reason, they are largely used in the investigation of basic cognitive processes.

It is possible to distinguish between early components linked to stimulus perception analysis, including the elaboration of physical features, referred to as *perceptual* or *exogenous potentials* or *early latency potentials*, and late components, related to cognitive operations (*cognitive* or *endogenous* or *long latency* potentials). More recently, this distinction has been replaced by a new classification that highlights differences between automatic early responses and cognitive strategic responses [45]. Moreover, ERPs can be classified by components with regard to their *polarity* (positive or negative), *amplitude*, and *latency* of insurgence (from stimulus onset).

The study of cognitive processes, involving amplitude and latency parameters, is based on the assumption that any cognitive process can be read as the addition of sequential (at times parallel) combinations of sub-processes. The organization of the sub-processes in sub-components may be considered an arbitrary subdivision that depends on the cognitive model adopted [46]. The hypothesis underlying the analysis of ERPs is that the transient electrical activity of brain potentials reflects the underlying nervous and cognitive processes involved in that task. Therefore, the spatial and temporal features of ERPs allow inferences to be drawn with respect to the cortical regions involved in those processes and the time-course of their basic components [47].

2.4.4.3
ERPs, Language, and Communication Studies

The study of language, including phonological, lexical, syntactic, and semantic processes, through ERPs has evidenced a distinction between the elaboration of verbs and nouns, the phonological *vs* acoustic elaboration of words, open and closed word classes, and further subdivision into syntactic and semantic elaborations [48, 49]. On a dynamic level, ERPs have been used to explore second-language acquisition and the development of linguistic and communicative competence from early age to adulthood. In this following, we present just a few of the possible applications of ERPs to the study of semantic elaboration (see Chapter 3).

For example, the N400 component is a negative deflection appearing about 400 ms after stimulus onset in posterior bilateral regions [50, 51] and is traditionally associated with semantic anomalies. The amplitude of the N400 effect appears to be a direct function of the grade of anomaly or stimulus incongruence with the context [52, 53]. Specifically, it seems to be an index of a more general stimulus-context incongruence, since it has been detected in relation to single words (word pairs, ambiguous words, words lists, etc.), as well as more complex sentences. More recently, it has been hypothesized that the N400 effect is linked to an individual's need to restore previous expectations on the level of semantic representation or, by contrast, to the cognitive effort demanded by elaboration processes for their assignment to working memory. The N400 is particularly relevant in the analysis of non-verbal components of communication in order to explore their relation to general communicative context. For instance, recent studies reported an N400 effect relative to non-standard meanings such as metaphor elaboration [54, 55]. Finally, studies focusing on the convergence and attuning of different non-verbal communication systems reported an increased N400 component in response to mismatching between vocal and mimic components in the communication of emotions [56].

2.4.4.4
Magnetoencephalography and Transcranial Magnetic Stimulation

In the previous paragraph, we described the measurement of time-by-time variations of brain activity associated with particular cognitive events through non-invasive recording at the scalp level. However, ERPs are unable to provide sufficiently precise information about the localization of neural activity sources. This limit is overcome by magnetoencephalography (MEG), which due to its non-invasiveness has been employed with increasing frequency in the study of language [57]. Moreover, MEG offers good resolution on both the spatial and the temporal level, although it records only superficial activity. Through appropriate sensors, MEG detects small variations of the magnetic field produced by neuronal electrical activity (tangential and radial fields), synchronized with external events. To measure the magnetic fields produced by small areas, MEG uses a neuromagnetometer. The signal/noise ratio is increased by recording multiple MEG responses to reiterated experimental events, thus obtaining an average profile of magnetic variations. For this reason, MEG indexes are referred to as evoked magnetic fields and they are the magnetic analogue of evoked potentials.

One of the most important advantages of MEG is the localization of cerebral activation sources connected to a specific event, in order to define architectural models of cognitive processes. However, the individuation of sources is extremely complex due, in the first place, to the difficulty of calculating the parameters of intracranial sources (spatial coordinates, strength and orientation of magnetic fields) starting from superficial measurement of the magnetic fields at the scalp surface. This problem is partially solved by the integration of MEG recordings with data from other systems, such as lesion studies by functional imaging techniques. In addition, powerful amplifying systems permit the mapping of magnetic field variations onto the anatomic image obtained through magnetic resonance imaging, providing a global image of the anatomic-functional characteristics of a certain area.

Another advantage of MEG is its better temporal resolution compared to other neuroimaging techniques. Moreover, MEG allows data interpretation in the absence of comparisons with data from other subjects in order to define the "average profile," which is necessary, for example, in functional magnetic resonance imaging. In other words, MEG combines the high temporal resolution typical of ERPs with the possibility of locating activity sources within sufficiently circumscribed brain regions.

Among the principal MEG studies applied to communication, Basile and colleagues [58] identified specific regions in the frontal cortex that are involved in the preparation and execution of different non-verbal operations. In addition, event-related magnetic fields (ERFs) were recorded by Sammelin and colleagues [59] in a study of word denomination.

Studies on complex cognitive processes have also been based on MEG. For example, a study on category discrimination for auditory stimuli (words) reported a bilateral negative deflection (N100), followed by a field with maximum amplitude around 400 ms (N400m) in the left hemisphere [60]. More recently, studies have tried to directly correlate ERPs and ERFs (such as N400 and N400m), reaching interesting conclusions (see [61] for an example).

Transcranial magnetic stimulation (TMS) is a recently developed technique that employs a magnetic field to influence language production processes [9]. This modern and non-invasive approach is based on the principle of electromagnetic induction, according to which an electric current flowing through a metallic coil generates a magnetic field vertically oriented to the electrical field. The coil is held to the scalp and connected to a capacitor. The electrical field generated induces a magnetic field of brief duration (about 180–300ms) that passes through the skin, muscles, and skull and reaches the cortex, where, under prolonged stimulation conditions, it temporally activates or inhibits the nearby cortical area. In communication studies, TMS permits interventions in speech production [62, 63, 64]. It is also used with the intent to stimulate the cortical areas of study participants [65].

2.4.5 Neuroimaging: Structural and Functional Techniques

The analytical study of cerebral activity has been facilitated by the improvement of bioimaging recording techniques [66]. Two different types of imaging techniques allow the investigation of different aspects of cognitive activity: *structural* imaging and *functional* imaging. Each method measures specific aspects of brain physiology, such as blood flow, oxygen and glucose metabolism, or the intracellular current of neurons. Imaging methods have allowed brain events within small anatomic regions to be individuated with extreme precision. Moreover, functional images are able to reflect cerebral operations and mechanisms, providing an index of the levels of activation of large populations of neurons. In other words, brain images reveal the activity of the architecture underlying the functional systems involved in communicative operations.

2.4.5.1 Structural Imaging

Within this category, two techniques have been extensively used clinically and experimentally: *computerized axial tomography* (CAT) and *nuclear magnetic resonance* (NMR). Both provide a structural but non-functional image of the brain [67]. Therefore, in the imaging of a damaged brain, all that can be seen is the macroscopic structural alteration, with no signs of the potential functional alteration caused by the lesion. Specifically, CAT is used to analyze brain structures in vivo as well as brain tissue density by measuring X-ray absorption values, with a gray scale representing the different levels of absorption. In NMR, a spectrometer creates magnetic fields of variable intensity. The technique exploits the properties of magnetic nuclei, which, when placed in a magnetic field and stimulated with electromagnetic pulses, radiate part of the energy absorbed in the form of radio signals. Studies of the behavior of these nuclei, including information related to the time they need to return to a normal state, may be used to reproduce the cortical anatomy. CAT images are typically bi-dimensional, whereas NMR images are tri-dimensional. Each element defining a point in space (defined by x and y coordinates) is called a *pixel*, while the element which defines a point in tri-dimensional space (coordinates x, y, z) is called a *voxel* (volumetric unit). In CAT and NMR images, pixels and voxels, respectively, are units that allow measurements of the structures depicted in the images.

2.4.5.2 Functional Imaging

Functional imaging is often employed in studying the neural basis of cognitive function, such as communication and language. In this paragraph, we focus on non-invasive measurement methods, such as those based on hemodynamic variations, i.e., *positron emission tomography* (PET) and *functional magnetic resonance imaging* (fMRI) (see [68]).

Both PET and fMRI are based on a direct relationship between changes in neuronal activity and blood flow modifications. Specifically, changes in blood flow and tissue metabolism within a specific brain area are assumed to be related to the activity performed by that area during the performance of a specific task. The greater the functional activity of an area of the brain, the higher its metabolic and blood flow

2

demands. Therefore, hemodynamic flow provides an indirect measure of increasing neural activity. It should be noted that blood flow changes occur only as a consequence of a change in the metabolic demand of neurons in general and not as a consequence of transient variations of single neurons (from asynchronous to synchronous), which would be of limited functional meaning. The most important hemodynamic measures and modalities are: tracking of *cerebral blood flow* (CBF), *single photon emission computed tomography* (SPECT), PET and fMRI.

Increases in blood supply to specific brain areas correlated to a specific task can be detected by measuring CBF. The technique involves the intracarotid injection of a radioactive isotope (xenon 133), followed by measurement of isotope distribution (variations of isotope concentration in time and distribution of the isotope in different brain areas) through the detection of gamma radiation. By correlating the results with morphological images obtained by CAT, it is possible to show that areas with altered blood perfusion are those involved by structural lesions. One of the most relevant contributions of the CBF technique has been the possibility to demonstrate that task-related performances do not involve a circumscribed brain region, but rather a distributed network of interconnected areas.

Computerized tomography monitors radioactive tracer distribution in a specific tissue, thus providing morphological and functional information. SPECT, through a rotating scanning system (gamma camera), allows CBF to be assessed in the form of gamma-ray emitting isotopes. Signals coming from the gamma camera are transformed by a computer into images similar to those provided by CAT, allowing the collection of morphological as well as functional data.

In the study of brain activity by PET, glucose metabolism is followed. The technique is based on the principle that any task makes energetic demands, thus increasing blood flow and metabolism. Finally, fMRI measures hemodynamic variations due to changes in neural activity during brain activities. Table 2.1 lists the advantages and disadvantages of the different functional imaging techniques.

Table 2.1 Strengths and weaknesses of electrophysiological and hemodynamic methods

	Strengths	Weaknesse
Electrophysiological	Direct measure of neural activity High temporal resolution Reliability of data relative to a specific performance	Partial samples of engaged functions Poor spatial resolution
Hemodynamic	Homogenous sampling (PET) or almost homogenous sampling (fMRI) of activations relative to a task High spatial resolution	Indirect measure of neural activity Low temporal resolution Difficulties in obtaining data relative to a specific performance Difficulties in distinguishing data relative to subject's state and to stimuli manipulation

Empirical studies using functional imaging technologies have redefined cortical maps in terms of the contribution of brain regions to specific linguistic and communicative functions, replacing the traditional model proposed by Broca-Wernicke (see [69] for a review). For instance, Petersen and colleagues [70] used PET to investigate word elaboration under three different conditions: word reading, the repetition of words aloud, and word-verb association. The three conditions were tested in auditory and visual modalities. The comparison of each condition with preceding levels through a "subtraction paradigm" resulted in different maps for the three different linguistic tasks.

In conclusion, electrophysiological and hemodynamic methodologies can be considered as complimentary instruments that, per se, are not able to provide complete representation of brain function. Images with high temporal and spatial resolution images must therefore be integrated in order to identify the fundamental structural and functional characteristics of linguistic and communicative processes.

References

1. Vallar G (2006) Metodi di indagine [Methods of analysis]. In: Cacciari C, Papagno C (eds) Psicologia generale e neuroscienze cognitive [General psychology and cognitive neuroscience]. Il Mulino, Bologna
2. Banich MT (1997) Neuropsychology: the neural bases of mental function. Houghton Mifflin, Boston
3. McCarthy RA, Warrington EK (1990) Cognitive neuropsychology: a clinical introduction. Academic Press, San Diego
4. Hellige JB (1998) Unity of language and communication: interhemispheric interaction in the lateralized brain. In: Stemmer B, Whitaker HA (eds) Handbook of neurolinguistics. Academic, San Diego, pp 405-414
5. Rugg MD (1999) Functional neuroimaging in cognitive neuroscience. In: Brown CM, Hagoort P (eds) The neurocognition of language. Oxford University Press, New York, pp 37-79
6. Fodor JA (1983) The modularity of mind. The MIT Press, Cambridge Mass
7. Shallice T (1988) From neuropsychology to mental structure. Cambridge University Press, Cambridge
8. Jackendoff R (2000) Fodorian modularity and representational modularity. In: Grodzinsky Y, Shapiro LP, Swinney D (eds) Language and the brain: representation and processes. Academic Press, San Diego, pp 3-30
9. Whitaker HA (1998) Neurolinguistics from the Middle Ages to the Pre-Modern era: historical vignettes. In: Stemmer B, Whitaker HA (eds) Handbook of neurolinguistics. Academic Press, San Diego, pp 27-54
10. Marraffa M, Meini C (2005) La mente sociale: le basi cognitive della comunicazione [The social mind: the cognitive bases of communication]. Laterza, Roma Bari
11. Aglioti SM, Fabbro F (2006) Neuropsicologia del linguaggio [Neuropsychology of language]. Il Mulino, Bologna
12. Johnston B, Stonnington HH (2009) Rehabilitation of neuropsychological disorders. A practical guide for rehabilitation professionals. Psychology Press, New York
13. Viggiano MP (2004) Valutazione cognitiva e neuropsicologica nel bambino, nell'adulto e nell'anziano [Cognitive and neuropsychological screening in childhood, adulthood, and old age]. Carocci, Roma

2

14. Commodari E (2002) Disturbi del linguaggio. I deficit della comunicazione orale: strumenti di valutazione e riabilitazione. Città Aperta, Enna
15. Lezak MD (1995) Neuropsychological assessment. Oxford University Press, New York
16. Spinnler H, Tognoni G (1987) Standardizzazione e taratura italiana di test neuropsicologici. Ital J Neurol Sci 6:suppl
17. Caramazza A, Hillis A (1989) The disruption of sentence production: some dissociations. Brain Lang 36:625-650
18. Carlomagno S, Labruna L, Blasi V (1998) La valutazione pragmatico-funzionale dei disturbi del linguaggio nel cerebroleso adulto [The pragmatic-functional screening of language deficits in brain damaged adults]. In: Carlomagno S, Caltagirone C (eds) La valutazione del deficit neurologico e comportamentale nella pratica neurologica. Global Services, London
19. Prutting C, Kirchner D (1987) A clinical appraisal of the pragmatics aspects of language. J Speech Hear Disord 52:105-119
20. Penn C (1988) The profiling of sintax and pragmatics in aphasia. Clin Linguist Phonet 2:179-207
21. Porch BE (1971) Porch Index of Communicative Ability. Vol 1. Theory and development. Consulting Psychology Press, Palo Alto
22. Porch BE (1981) Porch Index of Communicative Ability. Vol. 2. Administration, scoring and interpretation (3rd ed). Consulting Psychology, Palo Alto
23. Holland A (1980) Communicative abilities in daily living. University Park Press, Baltimora
24. Brookshire RH, Nicholas LE (1993) Discourse comprehension test. Communication Skill Builders, Tucson
25. Ekman P (1992) An argument for basic emotion. Cognition Emotion 6:169-200
26. Newport EL (1990) Maturational constraints on language learning. Cognitive Sci 14:11-28
27. Münte T, Heinze H (1994) Brain potentials reveal deficits of language processing after closed head injury. Arch Neurol-Chicago 51:482-493
28. Obler L, Fein D, Nicholas M, Albert M (1991) Auditory comprehension and aging: decline in syntactic processing. Appl Psycholinguis 12:433-452
29. Davidson R, Leslie S, Saron C (1990) Reaction time measures of interhemispheric transfer time in reading disabled and normal children. Neuropsychologia 28:471-485
30. Caplan D (1992) Language: structure, processing and disorders. The MIT Press, Cambridge
31. Arguin M, Bub D, Dudek G (1996) Shape integration for visual object recognition and its implication in category-specific visual agnosia. Vis Cogn 3:221-275
32. Chertkow H, Bub D, Bergman H et al (1994) Increased semantic priming in patients with dementia of the Alzheimer type. J Clin Exp Neuropsyc 16:608-622
33. Just M, Carpenter P (1993) The intensity dimension of thought: pupillometric indices of sentence processing. Can J Exp Psychol 47:310-339
34. Liversedge SP, Findlay JM (2000) Saccadic eye movements and cognition. Trends Cogn Sci 4:7-14
35. Balconi M (in press) Il comportamento visivo: elementi di psicologia e neuropsicologia dei movimenti oculari. [Eye-behavior. Psychology and Neuropsychology of Eye-movements]. Centro Scientifico Editore, Torino
36. Rayner K (1998) Eye movements in reading and information processing: 20 years of research. Psychol Bull 124:372-422
37. Andreassi JL (2000) Psychophysiology: human behavior and physiological response. Erlbaum, Mahwah
38. Öhman A, Hamm A, Hugdahl K (2000) Cognition and the autonomic nervous system: orienting, anticipation and conditioning. In: Cacioppo JT, Tassinary LG, Berntson GG (eds) Handbook of psychophysiology. Cambrige University Press, New York, pp 522-575
39. Cacioppo JT, Tassinary LG, Berntson GG (2000) Handbook of psychophysiology. Cambrige University Press, New York

40. Balconi M (2006) Neuropsychology and cognition of emotional face comprehension. Research Sign Post, Kerala
41. Balconi M, Mazza G (2009) Lateralisation effect in comprehension of emotional facial expression: a comparison between EEG alpha band power and behavioural inhibition (BIS) and activation (BAS) systems. Laterality 17:1-24
42. Moser JS, Haycak J, Bukay E, Simons RF (2006) Intentional modulation of emotional responding to unpleasant pictures: an ERP study. Psychophysiology 43:292
43. Cacioppo JT, Tassinary LG, Berntson GG (2000) Handbook of psychophysiology. Cambridge University Press, Cambridge
44. Handy TC (2005) Event-related potentials: a methods handbook. The MIT Press, Cambridge
45. Steinhauer K, Connolly JF (2008) Event-related potentials in the study of language. In: Stemmer B, Withaker HA (eds) Handbook of the neuroscience of language. Elsevier, Amsterdam, pp 91-103
46. Zani A, Mado Proverbio A (2000) Elettrofisiologia della mente. Carocci, Roma
47. Rugg MD, Coles MGH (1995) Electrophysiology of mind. Oxford University Press, Oxford
48. De Vincenzi M, Di Matteo R (2004) Come il cervello comprende il linguaggio [How brain understands language]. Laterza, Roma Bari
49. Segalowitz SJ, Chevalier H (1998) Event-related potential (ERP) research in neurolinguistics. Part II: Language processing and acquisition. In: Stemmer B, Whitaker HA (eds) Handbook of Neurolinguistics. Academic Press, San Diego, pp 111-123
50. Kutas M, Hillyard SA (1983) Event-related brain potentials to grammatical errors and semantica anomalies. Memory Cognition 11:539-550
51. Balconi M, Pozzoli U (2005) Comprehending semantic and grammatical violations in Italian. N400 and P600 comparison with visual and auditory stimuli. J Psycholinguist Res 34:71-98
52. Balconi M, Pozzoli U (2003) ERPs (event-related potentials), semantic attribution, and facial expressions of emotions. Conscious Emotion 4:63-80
53. Balconi M, Lucchiari C (2008) Consciousness and arousal effects on emotional face processing as revealed by brain oscillations. A gamma band analysis. Int J Psychophysiol 67:41-46
54. Tartter VC, Gomes H, Dubrovsky B et al (2002) Novel metaphors appear anomalous at least momentarily: evidence from N400. Brain Lang 80:488-509
55. Balconi M, Amenta S (2009) Pragmatic and semantic information interplay in ironic meaning computation: Evidence from "pragmatic-semantic" P600 effect. J Int Neuropsychol Soc 15:86
56. Balconi M (2008) Neuropsychology and psychophysiology of emotional face comprehension. Some empirical evidences. In: Balconi M (ed) Emotional face comprehension. Neuropsychological perspectives. Nova Science, New York, pp 23-57
57. Papanicolaou AC, Panagiotis GS, Basile LFH (1998) Applications of magnetoencephalography to neurolinguistic research. In: Stemmer B, Whitaker HA (eds) Handbook of neurolinguistics. Academic Press, San Diego, pp 143-158
58. Basile LFH, Rogers RL, Bourbon WT, Papanicolaou AC (1994) Slow magnetic fields from human frontal cortex. Electroen Clin Neuro 90:157-165
59. Salmelin R, Hari R, Lounasmaa OV, Sams M (1994) Dynamics of brain activation during picture naming. Nature 368:463-465
60. Hari R, Hämäläinen M, Kaukoranta E et al (1989) Selective listening modifies activity in the human auditory cortex. Exp Brain Res 74:463-470
61. Simos PJ, Basile LFH, Papanicolaou AC (1997) Source localization of the N400 response in a sentence-reading paradigm using evoked magnetic fields and magnetic resonance imaging. Brain Res 762:29-39
62. Pascual-Leone A, Grafman J, Clark K et al (1991) Procedural leariníng in Parkinson's disease and cerebellar degeneration. Ann Neurol 34:594-602

63. Stewart L, Walsh V, Frith U, Rothwell J (2001) Transcranial magnetic stimulation produces speech arrest but not song arrest. Ann NY Acad Sci 930:433-435
64. Manenti M, Cappa SF, Rossini PM, Miniussi C (2008) The role of prefrontal cortex in sentence comprehension: an rTMS study. Cortex 44:337-344
65. Cappa SF, Sandrini M, Rossini PM et al (2002) The role of the left frontal lobe in action naming: rTMS evidence. Neurology 59:720-723 6
66. Vallar G (2007) Gli esami strumentali nella neuropsicologia clinica [The strumental examinations of clinical neuropsychology]. In: Vallar G, Papagno C (eds) Manuale di neuropsicologia [Manual of neuropsychology]. Il Mulino, Bologna
67. Làdavas E, Berti AE (1995) Neuropsicologia [Neuropsychology]. Il Mulino, Bologna
68. Démonet JF (1998) Tomographic brain imaging of language functions: prospects for a new brain/language model. In: Stemmer B, Whitaker HA (eds) Handbook of neurolinguistics. Academic Press, San Diego, pp 132-143
69. Démonet JF, Thierry G, Cardebat D (2005) Renewal of the neurophysiology of language: functional neuroimaging. Physiol Rev 85:49-95
70. Petersen SE, Fox PT, Posner MI et al (1989) Positron emission tomographic studies of the processing of single words. J Cognitive Neurosci 1:153-170

Transcranial Magnetic Stimulation in the Study of Language and Communication

3

C. Miniussi, M. Cotelli, R. Manenti

3.1 Introduction

The results of many neuroimaging and high-resolution Electroencephalography (EEG) experiments, described in other chapters of this book, have revealed important correlative evidence for the involvement of several brain regions in linguistic communication. Neuroimaging and EEG techniques based on in vivo measurements of local changes in activity provide the best spatial and temporal resolution available. However, none of these techniques can unequivocally determine whether an active area is essential for a particular function or behavior [1].

Many lesion studies have reported the putative role of areas dedicated to the execution of cognitive tasks, and this approach is still very productive. Nevertheless, studies that attempt to infer normal function from single patients with brain damage are often criticized on the grounds that such cases provide evidence about the brain organization of a single individual but might not generalize to the rest of the population. A second criticism leveled at such studies is that chronic brain lesions can often lead to plastic changes that not only affect the region visibly damaged by the lesion but may also cause undamaged subsystems to be used in new ways. Therefore, the behavioral changes observed could reflect functional reorganization in the intact systems rather than loss of the damaged system. Thus, results from single cases, while extremely valuable, must always be interpreted with some caution, and it is important to obtain converging evidence using a variety of methods.

Transcranial magnetic stimulation (TMS) can be used to study the role of a particular brain region because it avoids the aforementioned criticisms. The use of TMS

C. Miniussi (✉)
Department of Biomedical Sciences and Biotechnologies, National Institute of Neuroscience, University of Brescia, Brescia; Cognitive Neuroscience Section, IRCCS San Giovanni di Dio Fatebenefratelli, Brescia, Italy

dates back to the mid-1980s, when Barker and colleagues [2] built the first magnetic stimulator able to non-invasively excite cortical neurons from the scalp surface. TMS is a tool that involves delivering a powerful (~2 T) and brief (~300 μs) magnetic pulse through a coil to the head of a participant. The magnetic field induces a brief electric current in the cortical surface under the coil, causing the depolarization of a population of cortical neurons. The TMS-induced activity in the subpopulation of neurons located under the stimulating coil interacts effectively with any pattern of activity that is occurring at the time of the stimulation [3]. Initial applications of TMS involved the delivery of single magnetic pulses. More recent technological advances allow the delivery of rhythmic trains of magnetic pulses, which is called repetitive TMS (rTMS).

There is general consensus that low-frequency rTMS consists of trains < 1 Hz, and high-frequency of rTMS trains > 5 Hz [4]. Treating low- and high-frequency rTMS as separate phenomena is essential, since these two kinds of stimulations might produce distinct effects on brain activity when applied offline for several minutes. Converging evidence indicates that rTMS < 1 Hz reduces cortical excitability both locally and in functionally related regions, while rTMS trains > 5 Hz seem to have opposite effects [5-7].

The use of rTMS in the field of cognitive neuroscience depends mainly on its ability to transiently interact with the stimulated cortical network, rather than on its modulation of cortical excitability. Therefore, rTMS application can be understood as two distinct approaches. Interaction with cognitive processing when rTMS is applied during performance of a task is called online TMS [3]. In contrast, in the case of offline stimulation, rTMS is applied for several minutes before the subject is tested on the task. Only in the latter case rTMS does affect the modulation of cortical excitability.

We now know more about some basic properties of TMS effects; these properties depend on the intensity (% of maximum stimulator output or % of motor threshold determined as the stimulation intensity necessary to produce a response of least 50 μV amplitude in a relaxed muscle in at least five out of ten consecutive stimulations [4]), frequency of stimulation (high *vs* low frequency), coil shape (focality, with the circular coil less focal than the figure-eight-shaped coil), orientation, and depth of stimulation, as well as the possible interactions between these factors. This basic knowledge is essential for planning TMS studies, but an adequate theoretical framework is also necessary for empirical data collection and interpretation [8].

In general, one of the great advantages of TMS is that it can be used in larger group of subjects, and the location of the coil can be precisely controlled with the neuronavigation approach. The second advantage is that TMS can be applied at different time points during the execution of a cognitive task, and thus it can also provide valuable information about when a brain region is involved in that task. Ultimately, in general, TMS could be used to map the flow of information across different brain regions during the execution of a complex cognitive task. Nevertheless, it should also be mentioned that, to date, even though the location of the stimulation can be precisely controlled, the spatial resolution of the induced effects is not yet fully clarified (see [9]). Therefore, sometimes the spatial resolution of rTMS effects hinders precise interpretation of the observed functional effects in terms of anatomical localization. A further problem of rTMS application might arise from the fact that the stimulating procedure is associated with a number of sensory perceptions (tactile and auditory). For instance, the discharging coil produces a click sound that may induce arousal and thereby disrupt task performance, irrespective of the exact demands of the experimental design. While this issue may be addressed by giving the subject earplugs to wear, such an approach is not practical for a language experiment requiring the subject to listen to voices or sounds. Finally, in all these experiments a control condition must be considered. Several approaches could be used to try to ensure that changes in performance are attributable specifically to the effects of TMS on the brain. One of these is sham stimulation, as a baseline condition. In the sham condition, the approach should ensure that no effective magnetic stimulation reaches the brain during the sham condition [10], while all the other experimental parameters are the same. Another approach is the stimulation of contralateral homologous areas (i.e., homotopic) while the subject performs the same task. This allows us to compare the effects of rTMS at different sites. Finally, it is also possible to observe subject behavior across several distinct tasks following stimulation at one site.

3.2 TMS and Language Studies

Language is a uniquely human ability that cannot be studied in animal models. Consequently, it is not surprising that TMS has been extensively applied to the study of the neural mechanisms of language, which cannot be investigated through the selective loss or gain of function in animal models. The TMS literature illustrates the difficulty in analyzing all aspects of language and the variability that characterizes most results (for a review, see [11]). Linguistic processing cannot be studied as a unique ability since it comprises a series of abilities that are quite diverse. The complexity of language indicates that research in this area might benefit from focusing on one aspect at a time. As a first subdivision, we could study language output (i.e., speech production) or input (i.e., speech comprehension), even though each of these abilities includes several different capacities. The following paragraphs present a brief summary of TMS studies of language.

3.2.1 Production

Speech production involves several cognitive processes [12]. The speaker has to choose the relevant information to be expressed, organize this information, and construct an ordered plan of what and how to speak (i.e., conceptual preparation). Then, the speaker has to select from the mental lexicon the adequate word forms to be used. These word forms also require syntactic ordering and correct grammatical inflection (i.e., grammatical encoding). Subsequently, the phonological forms of the words have to be retrieved from memory (i.e., lexical retrieval), and their syllabation, metrical structure, intonation, and articulatory motor commands have to be planned. Finally, these motor commands are executed, and overt speech is produced (i.e., articulation). Therefore, production involves several different processes (for a review, see [12]) that probably require different experimental paradigms and cognitive tasks for appropriate investigation (see other chapters in this book).

The rTMS-mediated interference of speech production was first examined at the beginning of the 1990s by Pascual-Leone et al. [13] in a population of epileptic patients awaiting surgery. The major aim of their study was to investigate the possibility of using rTMS as an alternative technique that could replace the invasive Wada test for determination of which hemisphere is dominant in language-related processes. The results showed that at high intensities of stimulation (80% of the stimulator output, circular coil, 8–25 Hz with a duration of 10 s), all subjects had total anarthria when rTMS was applied to the left frontotemporal region but not when it was placed above the right one, confirming left hemisphere dominance for language and, importantly, supporting concurrent Wada results. This effect has been called "speech arrest." The researchers [13] suggested that rTMS interfered specifically with language production and not simply with motor abilities necessary for speech output. These results were replicated by Jennum et al. [14], who studied epilepsy patients; complete speech arrest was described in 14 of 21 subjects. Interestingly, concordance with the Wada was 95%, and the subjects who did not report complete speech arrest found stronger stimulation too painful or could not be stimulated with higher intensities because the stimulator had already reached its maximum output. It is important to note that in this study the stimulation produced important contraction of facial and laryngeal muscles, leading also to dysarthria and creating problems for a clear interpretation of specific language difficulties [14, 15]. The main challenge in all of these studies is, therefore, the determination of whether effects are due to modulation of linguistic processes or to stimulation of the motor cortex/peripheral muscles. Most of the early studies with rTMS were limited to epilepsy patients because of concerns about the possibility of inducing seizures in normal subjects (see [4]) and because the aim was to compare rTMS data to the hemispheric language dominance for language determined by the Wada test. However, this population may not be representative of the normal population; thus, this choice may prevent generalization of the results. Anti-epileptic drugs were found to increase the intensity of stimulation needed to obtain an effect from rTMS. This change suggests that in these patients the "linguistic threshold" could be higher, resulting in less frequent production of the speech arrest than in healthy participants. Moreover, since the distribution of language areas in epilepsy patients might not be representative of that in normal subjects [16], the results obtained in this population may not be representative of those in healthy subjects.

Accordingly, the following studies on healthy subjects were performed over the last 15 years to more accurately localize the source of speech arrest among the normal population. First, Epstein et al. [17] reported that rTMS at lower frequencies required higher stimulator output but produced significantly less discomfort, together with less prominent contraction of facial musculature. Unlike a round stimulation coil, the coil used in that study (figure-eight-shaped) induced maximum electric fields beneath its center and more accurately identified the stimulated position. As these features have become increasingly precise, they have become more useful for determining the site of stimulation. Epstein et al. [18] suggested that some stimulation effects that had been previously ascribed to speech arrest (i.e., effect on language) could actually be due to motor cortex stimulation, but subsequently Stewart et al. [19] provided independent anatomical and physiological evidence of a dissociation between effects induced by frontal stimulation and pure motor effects following motor area stimulation. All these data identify the criteria necessary to define real speech arrest. The work of Stewart et al. [19] and Aziz-Zadeh et al. [20] showed that speech arrest can be induced by stimulation of two different sites within the frontal cortex; the authors were also able to attribute two different functional meanings to these two stimulation locations. When stimulating the more posterior site, stimulation of either the left or right hemisphere induced speech arrest; however, the effect was more evident with stimulation of the left hemisphere. Furthermore, stimulation at this site also evoked clear facial muscle contraction. In contrast, stimulation of the left and not the right anterior frontal cortex induced clear speech arrest; this type of stimulation did not evoke facial muscle contraction. These results led the authors to hypothesize that only stimulation of the more anterior site influences specific linguistic processes involved in speech production. In contrast, the stimulation of the more posterior site probably affects implementation of the motor sequence. These data clearly demonstrated the linguistic meaning of the speech arrest phenomenon.

Starting from these "localization" studies, other experiments were performed to investigate cortical functional subdivisions, particularly in the frontal cortex, depending on the specific linguistic ability to be studied. A representative case is the study of category-specific disorders that affect the subject's command of a grammatical class of words (nouns and verbs).

The problem of disorders selectively concerning nouns or verbs was raised by Goodglass et al [21], who were able to demonstrate opposite patterns of performance in patients with Broca's aphasia and those with fluent aphasia during naming tasks using pictures of objects and actions as stimuli. Broca's aphasics were mainly impaired in naming actions, whereas fluent aphasics showed a prevalent impairment in naming objects.

Damasio and co-workers hypothesized the existence of two-way-access systems that mediate a connection between concepts and word forms [22, 23], proposing that such systems for entities denoted by proper nouns are likely to be located in the left temporal pole, while mediation systems for certain categories of natural entities denoted by common nouns are located in left lateral and inferior temporal regions [24, 25]. On the other hand, Damasio and co-workers suggested that mediation systems for verbs could be located in frontal and parietal sites [24, 26].

Several clinical observations have suggested that different cerebral areas are involved in the processing of nouns and verbs. There is ample evidence that aphasic patients may be selectively impaired in the naming of objects or of actions. A double dissociation between object and action naming performance has been reported in individual cases [27, 28]. A difference in the cerebral localization of lesions has been suggested to underlie this behavioral dissociation; patients with a selective disorder for naming usually had lesions centered on the left temporal lobe. Conversely, selective impairment of action naming has been associated with large lesions usually extending to the left frontal cortex [29]. These observations have led to the hypothesis [22] that the neural networks subserving noun and verb retrieval are distinct, with left frontal convexity playing a crucial role in verb retrieval.

Shapiro et al. [30] used TMS to investigate functional specializations for distinct grammatical classes in the prefrontal cortex by stimulating the left prefrontal cortex during the production of nouns, verbs (e.g., "song" "songs" or "sing" "sings"), pseudonouns or pseudoverbs (e.g., "flonk"). Real and sham stimulation showed that response times following real stimulation increased for verbs and pseudoverbs but were unaffected for nouns and pseudonouns. Accordingly, it was suggested that grammatical categories have a neuroanatomical basis and that the left prefrontal cortex is selectively engaged in processing verbs as grammatical objects (i.e., effect on both verbs and pseudoverbs). Word production during speech is a multistage process with separate components involved in the computation of different aspects of the speech (meaning, grammatical function, sound, etc.), and each of these components could be mediated by different structures. Shapiro's data demonstrated for the first time that neural circuits in the left frontal cortex are particularly engaged in verb production and paved the way for study of the different processes involved in speech production, thus allowing differentiation of cortical areas that have different roles.

One task that could be used to investigate a specific aspect of speech production is picture naming. In the last 10 years, some studies have demonstrated interesting facilitative effects upon application of rTMS during picture-naming tasks. The facilitative results particularly evident with these kinds of tasks led to rehabilitation studies in patients reporting linguistic deficits. First, in healthy subjects, Topper et al. [31] studied the effects of TMS on picture-naming latencies by stimulating both the left motor region and Wernicke's area. TMS of the motor cortex had no effect, while stimulation of Wernicke's area significantly decreased picture-naming latencies, but only when stimulation was applied 500 and 1000 ms before picture presentation. Interestingly, the effects were present upon stimulation with an intensity of 35% or 55% of maximum stimulator output but disappeared with higher stimulation intensities. These data suggest that focal TMS facilitates lexical processes, likely inducing a general pre-activation of linguistic neural networks even if the bases of these effects are not yet clear.

We have therefore used online rTMS to transiently modulate the neural circuitry involved in picture naming in two groups of subjects. In the first study, rTMS was applied to dorsolateral prefrontal cortices (DLPFCs) in three experimental blocks (rTMS to the right and left DLPFC, and sham stimulation) in healthy volunteers. The subjects were instructed to name the picture as quickly as possible and trains of rTMS (500 ms, 20 Hz) were delivered simultaneously with picture presentation. We found a selective facilitation during action naming when the subjects received stimulation to the left DLPFC, as compared to the right DLPFC and sham conditions [32]. Object naming was not affected. These facilitative results encouraged a second study evaluating the possibility of increasing performance in a patient sample [33]. We applied the same experimental paradigm (i.e., object- and action-naming tasks and rTMS of DLPFC) to fifteen probable Alzheimer's disease (AD) patients. As word-finding difficulty (anomia) is commonly present in the early stages of AD, the aim of the study was to assess whether rTMS could improve naming performance. We found that action-naming performance was significantly improved during rTMS applied to the left and right DLPFC (mean 17%), as compared to sham stimulation. Moreover, the improvement was present in all subjects, whereas object naming was unaffected by the stimulation. Subsequently, we applied the same paradigm to a group of 24 probable AD patients with different degrees of cognitive decline. As previously reported, stimulation of both the left and the right DLPFC improved action but not object naming in the mild AD group. Improved naming accuracy for both classes of stimuli was found in the moderate to severe group [34]. This study allowed us to confirm that rTMS applied to the DLPFC improves naming performance in the advanced stages of AD and to show that in the severe group the effect is not specific for action naming. We suggest that this methodology can affect the intrinsic ability of the brain to restore or compensate for damaged function and may represent a useful new tool for cognitive rehabilitation. Although the effect on action naming was quite robust, the underlying mechanisms remain unclear, and the basis for the facilitative effects of rTMS on lexical retrieval is uncertain. Future studies using a combination of stimulation and imaging techniques could determine whether and how behavioral facilitation is mediated by cortical changes and if this could be a useful complementary technique in the treatment of language dysfunctions in aphasic patients [35].

3.2.2 Comprehension

The ability to produce and understand sentences requires the computation of syntactic structures and is frequently affected by neurological damage. Typically, patients with focal brain damage involving Broca's area show agrammatism in production (i.e., they tend to produce short, syntactically simplified sentences with reduced morphology) and are often impaired in the comprehension of syntactically complex sentences (see [36] for a review). In addition, the deceptively simple act of understanding the meaning of a common sentence included in speech requires a number of cognitive processes. Minimally, these include the analysis of phonological and syntactic structures, as well as of the meaning of the lexical items. Sentence comprehension requires processing a sequence of words as well as analyzing their syntactic and thematic organization to create a correct representation of the entire sentence. This elaboration requires the maintenance of an activated state of both single-word meaning and the syntactic relations between words [37]. While current models of language comprehension make different predictions with regard to the proposed time course of syntactic and semantic integration, there is general agreement that these processes require the temporary storage and manipulation of multiple classes of information [38]. Both storage and manipulation are thought to depend upon working memory (WM) resources.

The complexity of speech comprehension processes and the continuous integration of linguistic and memory processes in comprehension tasks (such as sentence judgments or reading) create several difficulties in the study of TMS effects on comprehension. To date, only a few studies have been reported.

Effects on language comprehension are difficult to obtain using both single-pulse and repetitive TMS. Even with rTMS above temporal and parietal areas, Claus et al. [39] showed no effects on three-syllable and six-digit readings. The authors were, however, able to show significant hemispheric differences exclusively in the reading of four-word sentences. Sentences were displayed on a computer screen for an interval brief enough that, at baseline, 10–50% of words were reported incorrectly. rTMS was then administered simultaneously with sentence presentation. Subjects made significantly more errors with left-sided stimulation, but only on the most difficult types of sentences and exclusively in subjects who used "an integral strategy of reading" and in "pure" right-handers who reported that they did not have left-handed relatives. The possibility of interference occurring only when using longer and more difficult items again suggests a possible influence of memory resources on the linguistic task because the reading of four-word sentences more likely requires memory processes than the reading of three syllables.

Another way to study linguistic comprehension is to start from words (i.e., included in the sentences that compose speech) and investigate effects on lexical decision tasks, which necessarily involve a comprehension of the presented items, using words of different categories (e.g., abstract and concrete words). Recently, the processing of abstract/concrete nouns using rTMS and a lexical decision paradigm was studied [40]. Interference with accuracy was found for abstract words when rTMS was applied over the left superior temporal gyrus, while for concrete words, accuracy decreased when rTMS was applied over the right contralateral homologous site. Moreover, accuracy for abstract words, but not for concrete words, decreased after left frontal inferior gyrus stimulation. These results suggest that abstract lexical entries are stored in the posterior part of the left temporal and possibly in the left frontal sites, while the regions involved in storing concrete items include the right temporal cortex.

An interesting study on sentence judgment was conducted by Sakai and co-workers [41], who investigated whether Broca's area was involved in syntactic processing by using a sentence validation task. Participants viewed sentences and had to identify each sentence as correct or as grammatically or semantically incorrect. All sentences used a simple noun phrase-verb phrase (NP-VP) construction, with the VP appearing 200 ms after the NP. TMS to Broca's area was delivered at different time points after the VP: 0, 150, or 350 ms after the VP onset. Relative to sham stimulation, TMS selectively facilitated response times for syntactic, but not semantic, decisions, and the effect was evident exclusively when stimulation was applied 150 ms after VP onset. The results of this study suggest that Broca's area is causally involved in syntactic processing and that the function of this area is important for syntactic processing only 150 ms after VP onset. It is interesting to highlight the importance of this study in the context of the chronometry of linguistic processes. The authors were able to investigate the precise moment at which the target area was relevant for the studied process, including different possible time-windows in which stimulation could be applied.

The task used in this study required an explicit elaboration of the sentence in order to render an explicit judgment regarding structure/meaning. It could be important to understand what happens when the task is more implicit and thus more similar to daily living communication. This is called "online sentence comprehension," and in these tasks it has been reported to represent the crucial importance of Broca's area not only for syntactic integration [41] but also for WM mechanisms relevant for language processing [42]. The two factors of syntactic complexity and sentence length have often been confounded [39], and some imaging investigations have supported the view that inferior frontal gyrus activation is specific for syntactic processing, while engagement of the DLPFC may reflect the WM load [43-45]. A recent functional magnetic resonance imaging (fMRI) study, which analyzed the areas involved in a sentence judgment task, underlined the recruitment of the dorsal portion of the left frontal cortex. Specifically, this area is involved in the processing of syntactic violations associated with a large WM load [46], highlighting again the continuous integration of memory and language processes in speech comprehension.

In order to study speech comprehension more implicitly, a task called the sentence-picture matching task can be used. In this task, the meaning of the displayed sentence has to be clear to the participant in order for the participant to provide the correct response; however, the participant is not required to directly judge the sentence. Using rTMS, we investigated the role of the DLPFC in sentence comprehension using a sentence-picture matching task [47]. Given two pictures, subjects were required to choose the one that correctly matched the meaning of active and passive semantically reversible sentences (subject-verb-object); the incorrect picture did not match the sentence in terms of lexical items (semantic task) or agent–patient structure (syntactic task). The subjects performed the task while a series of magnetic stimuli were applied to the left or right DLPFC; an additional sham stimulation condition was included. When rTMS was applied to the left DLPFC, the subjects' performance was delayed only for the semantic task, whereas rTMS applied to the right DLPFC slowed the processing of syntactic information. The results of this experiment provide direct evidence of a double dissociation between the rTMS effects and the type of task. This may reflect a differential hemispheric involvement of WM resources during sentence comprehension, since verbal WM (i.e., left interference) would be involved in the semantic task while visual WM (i.e., right interference) would be important during the syntactic task [47]. This study is important because it provides direct proof of the critical involvement of WM processes in speech comprehension and further highlights the complexity of this deceptively simple act of daily life.

3.3
Motor Area and Language

Consistent evidence indicates a functional link between the motor area and language [48-51] and has encouraged TMS studies on this interesting relationship. Tokimura et al. [52] investigated the enhancement of motor responses from hand muscles during speech production. They recorded from the first finger (dorsal interosseus) of both hands during relaxation while subjects performed a variety of speech output tasks. Spontaneous speech increased the size of electromyography (EMG) responses bilaterally, whereas reading aloud increased EMG potentials only on one side, probably due to language-related hemisphere dominance. It was suggested that reading aloud increases excitability of the motor hand area in the dominant hemisphere and that this procedure might represent a simpler and safer alternative to the Wada test for assessment of cerebral dominance. It has been suggested that this link may reflect the irrepressible use of hand gestures when speaking, even if fMRI (for a particular example regarding listening, see [53, 54]) and rTMS have been used to study linguistic tasks that do not involve any production of movement [55-57]. In a recent effort to investigate the topographic localization of these effects, Fadiga and co-workers [58] found that auditory presentation of specific phonemes facilitated motor excitability measured from specific tongue muscles used in the production of those specific phonemes. Although it may seem obvious that speech production affects motor system excitability, it is potentially surprising that speech perception (i.e., listening) should also have this effect. Furthermore, taking advantage of the recently developed ability to combine TMS with imaging techniques, Watkins and Paus [59] investigated the brain regions that mediate the reported change in motor excitability during speech perception. Motor excitability induced by TMS was recorded over the facial area of the left motor cortex by eliciting motor-evoked potentials from the orbicularis oris muscle during auditory speech perception. These excitability measures were correlated with simultaneous regional cerebral blood flow (positron emission tomography data) across the entire brain. Increased motor excitability during speech perception correlated with increased blood flow in the posterior part of the left inferior frontal gyrus, the human homologue of the region containing mirror neurons in the macaque [60]. In other words, the combination of TMS with an imaging technique allowed researchers to prove that Broca's area plays a central role in linking speech perception with speech production, consistent with theories that emphasize the integration of sensory and motor representations in the understanding of speech [61, 62].

The results of all these studies support the notion that passive speech perception induces the activation of further brain areas involved in speech production. It has been proposed that the increased motor excitability of the speech production areas reflect covert imitative mechanisms, which may have enhanced speech comprehension abilities over the course of evolution (for a review, see [11]).

3.4 Conclusions

Clearly, TMS provides a non-invasive tool that allows the investigation of the neuronal basis of language in normal subjects. Its spatial and temporal resolution facilitates the search for answers to two important questions in cognitive neuroscience:

Which information is processed in a given brain structure? And when does this processing occur? [3]. Accordingly, TMS has been used to establish causality in brain-behavior relationships. Therefore, among the methodologies that neuroscientists can use to investigate the "working brain," TMS represents a unique and useful tool for the study of language.

References

1. Price CJ, Friston KJ (1999) Scanning patients with tasks they can perform. Hum Brain Mapp 8:102-108
2. Barker AT, Jalinous R, Freeston IL (1985) Non-invasive magnetic stimulation of human motor cortex. Lancet 1:1106-1107
3. Walsh V, Pascual-Leone A (2003) Transcranial magnetic stimulation: a neurochronometrics of mind. MIT Press Cambridge, MA
4. Rossi S, Hallett M, Rossini PM et al (2009) Safety, ethical considerations, and application guidelines for the use of transcranial magnetic stimulation in clinical practice and research. A consensus statement from the international workshop on "Present and future of TMS: Safety and ethical guidelines". Clin Neurophysiol 120:2008-2039
5. Maeda F, Keenan JP, Tormos JM et al (2000) Modulation of corticospinal excitability by repetitive transcranial magnetic stimulation. Clin Neurophysiol 111:800-805
6. Pascual-Leone A, Valls-Sole J, Wassermann EM, Hallett M (1994) Responses to rapid-rate transcranial magnetic stimulation of the human motor cortex. Brain 117:847-858
7. Chen R, Classen J, Gerloff C et al (1997) Depression of motor cortex excitability by low-frequency transcranial magnetic stimulation. Neurology 48:1398-1403
8. Miniussi C, Ruzzoli M, Walsh V (2010) The mechanism of transcranial magnetic stimulation in cognition. Cortex 46:128-130
9. Bestmann S, Ruff CC, Blankenburg F et al (2008) Mapping causal interregional influences with concurrent TMS-fMRI. Exp Brain Res 191:383-402
10. Rossi S, Ferro M, Cincotta M et al (2007) A real electro-magnetic placebo (remp) device for sham transcranial magnetic stimulation (TMS). Clin Neurophysiol 118:709-716
11. Devlin JT, Watkins KE (2007) Stimulating language: insights from TMS. Brain 130:610-622
12. Butterworth B (1980) Some constraints on models of language production. In: Butterworth B (ed) Language production, vol. 1. Speech and talk. Academic, London
13. Pascual-Leone A, Gates JR, Dhuna A (1991) Induction of speech arrest and counting errors with rapid-rate transcranial magnetic stimulation. Neurology 41:697-702
14. Jennum P, Friberg L, Fuglsang-Frederiksen A, Dam M (1994) Speech localization using repetitive transcranial magnetic stimulation. Neurology 44:269-273
15. Jennum P, Winkel H (1994) Transcranial magnetic stimulation. Its role in the evaluation of patients with partial epilepsy. Acta Neurol Scand Suppl 152:93-96
16. Woods RP, Dodrill CB, Ojemann GA (1988) Brain injury, handedness, and speech lateralization in a series of amobarbital studies. Ann Neurol 23:510-518
17. Epstein CM, Lah JJ, Meador K et al (1996) Optimum stimulus parameters for lateralized suppression of speech with magnetic brain stimulation. Neurology 47:1590-1593
18. Epstein CM (1999) Language and TMS/rTMS. Electroencephalogr Clin Neurophysiol Suppl 51:325-333
19. Stewart L, Walsh V, Frith U, Rothwell JC (2001) TMS produces two dissociable types of speech disruption. Neuroimage 13:472-478

3

20. Aziz-Zadeh L, Cattaneo L, Rochat M, Rizzolatti G (2005) Covert speech arrest induced by rTMS over both motor and nonmotor left hemisphere frontal sites. J Cogn Neurosci 17:928-938
21. Goodglass H, Klein B, Carey P, Jones K (1966) Specific semantic word categories in aphasia. Cortex 2:74-89
22. Damasio AR, Tranel D (1993) Nouns and verbs are retrieved with differently distributed neural systems. Proc Natl Acad Sci USA 90:4957-4960
23. Damasio H, Grabowski TJ, Tranel D et al (2001) Neural correlates of naming actions and of naming spatial relations. Neuroimage 13:1053-1064
24. Damasio AR, Damasio H (1992) Brain and language. Sci Am 267:88-95
25. Damasio AR, Damasio H, Tranel D, Brandt JP (1990) Neural regionalization of knowledge access: preliminary evidence. Cold Spring Harbor Symp Quant Biol 55:1039-1047
26. Damasio AR, Tranel D, Damasio H (1992) Verbs but not nouns: damage to left temporal cortices impairs access to nouns but not verbs. Soc Neurosci Abstract 18:387
27. Miceli G, Silveri MC, Nocentini U, Caramazza A (1988) Patterns of dissociation in comprehension and production of nouns and verbs. Aphasiology 2:351-358
28. Miozzo A, Soardi M, Cappa SF (1994) Pure anomia with spared action naming due to a left temporal lesion. Neuropsychologia 32:1101-1109
29. Daniele A, Giustolisi L, Silveri MC et al (1994) Evidence for a possible neuroanatomical basis for lexical processing of nouns and verbs. Neuropsychologia 32:1325-1341
30. Shapiro KA, Pascual-Leone A, Mottaghy FM et al (2001) Grammatical distinctions in the left frontal cortex. J Cogn Neurosci 13:713-720
31. Topper R, Mottaghy FM, Brugmann M et al (1998) Facilitation of picture naming by focal transcranial magnetic stimulation of Wernicke's area. Exp Brain Res 121:371-378
32. Cappa SF, Sandrini M, Rossini PM et al (2002) The role of the left frontal lobe in action naming: rTMS evidence. Neurology 59:720-723
33. Cotelli M, Manenti R, Cappa SF et al (2006) Effect of transcranial magnetic stimulation on action naming in patients with Alzheimer disease. Arch Neurol 63:1602-1604
34. Cotelli M, Manenti R, Cappa SF et al (2008) Transcranial magnetic stimulation improves naming in Alzheimer disease patients at different stages of cognitive decline. Eur J Neurol 15:1286-1292
35. Miniussi C, Cappa SF, Cohen LG et al (2008) Efficacy of repetitive transcranial magnetic stimulation/transcranial direct current stimulation in cognitive neurorehabilitation. Brain Stimulation 1:326-336
36. Grodzinsky Y (2000) The neurology of syntax: language use without Broca's area. Behav Brain Sci 23:1-71
37. Just MA, Carpenter PA (1992) A capacity theory of comprehension: individual differences in working memory. Psychol Rev 99:122-149
38. Friederici AD, Kotz SA (2003) The brain basis of syntactic processes: functional imaging and lesion studies. Neuroimage 20 Suppl 1:S8-17
39. Claus D, Weis M, Treig T et al (1993) Influence of repetitive magnetic stimuli on verbal comprehension. J Neurol 240:149-150
40. Papagno C, Fogliata A, Catricala E, Miniussi C (2009) The lexical processing of abstract and concrete nouns. Brain Res 1263:78-86
41. Sakai KL, Noguchi Y, Takeuchi T, Watanabe E (2002) Selective priming of syntactic processing by event-related transcranial magnetic stimulation of broca's area. Neuron 35:1177-1182
42. Fiebach CJ, Schlesewsky M, Lohmann G et al (2005) Revisiting the role of broca's area in sentence processing: syntactic integration versus syntactic working memory. Hum Brain Mapp 24:79-91

43. Caplan D, Vijayan S, Kuperberg G et al (2002) Vascular responses to syntactic processing: Event-related fMRI study of relative clauses. Hum Brain Mapp 15:26-38
44. Hashimoto R, Sakai KL (2002) Specialization in the left prefrontal cortex for sentence comprehension. Neuron 35:589-597
45. Walsh V, Rushworth M (1999) A primer of magnetic stimulation as a tool for neuropsychology. Neuropsychologia 37:125-135
46. Cooke A, Grossman M, DeVita C et al (2006) Large-scale neural network for sentence processing. Brain Lang 96:14-36
47. Manenti R, Cappa SF, Rossini PM, Miniussi C (2008) The role of the prefrontal cortex in sentence comprehension: an rTMS study. Cortex 44:337-344
48. Meister IG, Boroojerdi B, Foltys H et al (2003) Motor cortex hand area and speech: Implications for the development of language. Neuropsychologia 41:401-406
49. Lo YL, Fook-Chong S, Lau DP, Tan EK (2003) Cortical excitability changes associated with musical tasks: a transcranial magnetic stimulation study in humans. Neurosci Lett 352:85-88
50. Salmelin R, Sams M (2002) Motor cortex involvement during verbal versus non-verbal lip and tongue movements. Hum Brain Mapp 16:81-91
51. Saarinen T, Laaksonen H, Parviainen T, Salmelin R (2006) Motor cortex dynamics in visuomotor production of speech and non-speech mouth movements. Cereb Cortex 16:212-222
52. Tokimura H, Tokimura Y, Oliviero A et al (1996) Speech-induced changes in corticospinal excitability. Ann Neurol 40:628-634
53. Tettamanti M, Buccino G, Saccuman MC et al (2005) Listening to action-related sentences activates fronto-parietal motor circuits. J Cogn Neurosci 17:273-281
54. Tettamanti M, Manenti R, Della Rosa PA et al (2008) Negation in the brain: modulating action representations. Neuroimage 43:358-367
55. Watkins KE, Strafella AP, Paus T (2003) Seeing and hearing speech excites the motor system involved in speech production. Neuropsychologia 41:989-994
56. Sundara M, Namasivayam AK, Chen R (2001) Observation-execution matching system for speech: a magnetic stimulation study. Neuroreport 12:1341-1344
57. Aziz-Zadeh L, Iacoboni M, Zaidel E et al (2004) Left hemisphere motor facilitation in response to manual action sounds. Eur J Neurosci 19:2609-2612
58. Fadiga L, Craighero L, Buccino G, Rizzolatti G (2002) Speech listening specifically modulates the excitability of tongue muscles: a TMS study. Eur J Neurosci 15:399-402
59. Watkins K, Paus T (2004) Modulation of motor excitability during speech perception: the role of broca's area. J Cogn Neurosci 16:978-987
60. Kohler E, Keysers C, Umilta MA et al (2002) Hearing sounds, understanding actions: action representation in mirror neurons. Science 297:846-848
61. Hickok G, Poeppel D (2000) Towards a functional neuroanatomy of speech perception. Trends Cogn Sci 4:131-138
62. Scott SK, Wise RJ (2004) The functional neuroanatomy of prelexical processing in speech perception. Cognition 92:13-45

Electromagnetic Indices of Language Processing

4

A. Mado Proverbio, A. Zani

4.1 Models of Language Comprehension and Production

In this chapter, we describe the processes underlying language comprehension, both in the visual modality of reading and in the auditory modality of listening, by focusing on the main stages of linguistic information processing, from the sensory to the symbolic levels. Given the particular nature of the research techniques used, linguistic production mechanisms will not be addressed here, because of the well-known motor-related electromagnetic artifacts induced by spontaneous speech. Briefly, linguistic production mechanisms are based on the ability to: formulate a thought by accessing conceptual representations, provide it with a correct structure from the lexical (semantics) and syntactic points of view (ordering and attribution of roles), access the phonologic and phonemic form of the various discourse parts (nouns, verbs, function words), pre-program the muscular and articulatory movements involved in phonation, and implement those commands by performing the emission of appropriate linguistic phonemes fluently and with the right prosody.

Neurologic data on patients with unilateral focal lesions in different regions of the brain indicate the base of the third left frontal circumvolution as the area devoted to fluent language production and phonemic articulation (and whose damage results in Broca's aphasia), according to the Wernicke-Lichteim-Geschwind model. The area devoted to language comprehension, and to the representation of auditory forms of words, lies in the temporal cortex (whose damage results in Wernicke's aphasia). The area containing conceptual representations (necessary for spontaneous speech and word comprehension, but not for passive repetition of heard auditory inputs) lies in the angular and supramarginal gyrus of the parietal cortex. The arcu-

A. Mado Proverbio (✉)
Department of Psychology, University of Milano-Bicocca, Milan, Italy

Neuropsychology of Communication. Michela Balconi (Ed.)

ate fasciculus interconnects Broca's area with that of Wernicke, whose interruption results in conduction aphasia, characterized by the inability to repeat heard auditory material.

The mechanisms of written-word comprehension have been widely investigated by many researchers. In cognitive studies of language, usually the experimental paradigms involve the visual presentation of linguistic stimuli, including:

- words, which can vary as a function of their frequency of use, concreteness/abstractness, imagery value, and length; for example: ORANGE;
- pseudo-words, which are meaningless letter strings assembled according to the orthographic rules of the language (named "legal"); for example: MORLIENT;
- illegal strings, which are letter strings assembled without respecting concatenation rules; for example: PQERLZFQ;
- false characters, which are strings of non-linguistic symbols that can resemble (or not) real alphabetic characters; for example: ↓■➰♍⌖✍●.

According to the so-called two-way reading model of Coltheart [1], the processing of a linguistic visual stimulus can be carried out via activation of a *lexical route*, based on the global and immediate recognition of familiar stimuli, or a *phonologic route*, based on grapheme-to-phoneme conversion. It has been hypothesized that high-frequency words are directly recognized as unitary visual entities, whereas pseudo-words and low-frequency words are processed via the phonologic route. The existence of distinct reading pathways is supported by the evidence of patients with focal lesions that result in dissociation, and thus with specific impairment of one of the reading modalities. Coltheart's reading model has been successively modified to include a third, direct (non-semantic) route, which has been inserted in order to explain reading processes in hyperlexic patients. Such patients show accurate reading ability but without comprehension.

According to the standard model, the first stage of processing in reading consists of the sensory visual processing of letter strings and their physical characteristics (luminance, size, color, shape, orientation), followed by the gradual recognition of single letters. From this level, three routes of processing depart in parallel: the visual route, the phonologic route, and the direct route. In the lexical route, visual recognition of a stimulus takes place through access to the orthographic visual input. From there, it is possible to access the semantic system that stores word meanings. The first stage of the phonologic route allows access to the phonologic forms of inputs (strings, pseudo-words, or low-frequency words) according to the grapheme-to-phoneme conversion rules of the specific language. The main reading disabilities observed by neuropsychologists have been interpreted as specific impairments of the various reading pathways postulated by the standard model of reading. In particular, surface dyslexia, described by Marshall and Newcombe [2], which is more readily found in shallow languages such as English than in transparent languages such as Spanish or Italian, is characterized by regularization of irregular words (in transparent languages they consist of the incorrect attribution of accent) or by failures to perform the silent homophony test: for example, words having different visual forms but similar phonologic forms cannot be distinguished (in Italian, patients have trouble in discriminating between L'AGO (*needle*) and LAGO (*lake*). Superficial dyslexics behave as if they were unable to recognize words at first glance, and when they read they apply grapheme-to-phoneme conversion rules for each word. This clinical picture can be explained in terms of an impairment of the lexical route. Due to this interruption, patients read both words and non-words via the phonologic route by applying grapheme-to-phoneme transformation rules. This type of dyslexia, if acquired after a lesion or a trauma, is often associated with a left temporal lesion.

By contrast, phonologic dyslexia, described, for example, by Temple and Marshall [3], generally consists in the inability to read non-words, unknown non-words, and function words (and, if, for, in, on, etc.) while the ability to read words that are part of the usual vocabulary of the patient is preserved. This pattern can be explained by assuming an impairment of the phonologic route. Consequently, patients are able to recognize familiar words through the lexical route, but they are not able to apply the grapheme-to-phoneme conversion rules for items not visually recognized as familiar. Often, patients suffering from phonologic dyslexia have left occipito-parietal lesions, including the angular gyrus, which is involved in grapheme/phoneme mapping (see Par. 4.4).

4.2 Electrophysiology of Language

Figure 4.1 shows the time course of linguistic information processing based on data derived from the use of recording techniques of brain-evoked electromagnetic activity (event-related potentials, ERP, and magnetoencephalography, MEG). In particular, ERPs represent a unique tool in the study and analysis of different stages of linguistic information processing, since they are characterized, on the one hand, by the lack of invasiveness typical of electroencephalographic (EEG) recording, and, on the other hand, by an optimal temporal resolution (which may be < 1 ms).

The spatial resolution of ERPs is also good, especially when used in combination with techniques for the intracortical localization of neural generators, such as LORETA (low-resolution electromagnetic tomography), dipole modeling, MUSIC (multiple signal classification), and BESA (brain electric source analysis) or with functional magnetic resonance imaging (fMRI) data (Fig. 4.1).

While the origins and characteristics of the electromagnetic signal are treated in a more detailed manner elsewhere [4, 5], it is important to recall here that ERPs are obtained by averaging hundreds of EEG sweeps in order to amplify the tiny evoked signal hidden among large-voltage spontaneous EEG oscillations and which are relative to the specific nature of the cerebral processing in response to a given stimulus/event. The temporal latency onset of a given deflection or peak (positive or negative voltage shift) visible in the waveform of the evoked potential therefore represents the occurrence of brain processing activity time-locked to the event. For example, the occurrence of a potential variation at about 70–80 ms over the primary visual cortex indexes the arrival of incoming information to the visual cortex and the corresponding activation of neural populations involved in stimulus sensory processing

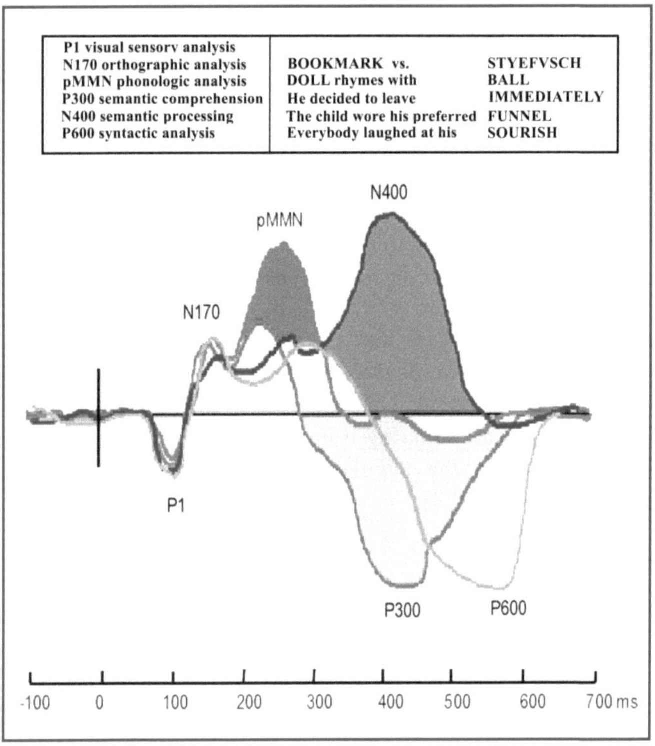

Fig. 4.1 Time course of cerebral activation during the processing of linguistic material, as reflected by the latency of occurrence of various ERP components. Pre-linguistic stimulus sensory processing occurs (P1 component) at about 100 ms post-stimulus; orthographic analysis of written words (posterior N1 component) at 150–200 ms; phonologic/phonetic analysis at 200–300 ms, as evidenced by phonological mismatch negativity (temporal and anterior pMMN) in response to phonologic incongruities (both visual and auditory); and a large centroparietal negativity at about 400 ms (N400), in response to semantic incongruities and indexing lexical access mechanisms. The comprehension of meaningful sentences reaches consciousness between 300 and 500 ms (P300 component); finally, a second-order syntactic analysis is indicated by the appearance of a late positive deflection (P600) at about 600 ms post-stimulus latency

(BA 17). In the same way, the occurrence of a large negative deflection at about 400 ms in response to semantically incomprehensible stimuli leads to semantic meaning analysis processes for a given word.

Thus, ERPs provide an important approach to analyzing the neural mechanisms enabling spoken language comprehension and silent reading, whereas verbal production mechanisms are hardly observable by means of EEG, since every muscular movement (such as those involved in phonation and speech) produce an electromyographic signal of considerable amplitude, which masks any variation in the synchronized cortical voltage. Surface cerebral bioelectric signals originate from extracellular excitatory and inhibitory post-synaptic potentials of neural populations that, besides being

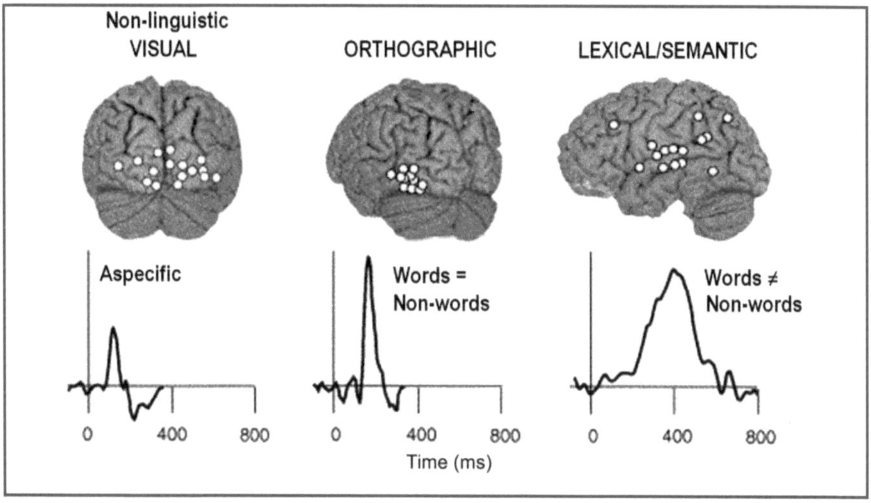

Fig. 4.2 Correspondence between the peak of event-related magnetic responses and the localization of intracortical generator. On the left, a non-specific sensory visual response is seen at about 100 ms of latency post-stimulus, involving the occipital cortex. In the middle, there is a negative peak of around 170 ms, which indicates probable activation of the left fusifom area, devoted to orthographic analysis. On the right, a large negative response reflects unsuccessful semantic recognition of non-words compared to existing words (around 400 ms), by the temporo-parietal cortex. (Modified from Salmelin [6], copyright (2007), with the permission of the International Federation of Clinical Neurophysiology)

synchronously active, are associated with apical dendrites perpendicularly oriented to the recording surface (EEG) or parallel to it (MEG). For MEG, optimal spatial resolution, reflecting magnetic field variations induced by bioelectrical dipoles and orthogonal to them, derives from the fact that magnetic signals are not subject to distortions while passing through the various tissues, i.e., gray and white matter, liquor, membranes, meninges, and skull, such that a clear correspondence is maintained between the intra-cortical generator and the surface distribution (Fig. 4.2).

ERP recording in the study of language comprehension mechanisms was applied for the first time at the end of 1970s by many researchers working in the field of what has since become known as Cognitive Neuroscience. In 1968, Sutton discovered that the human brain emitted a large positive response to those stimuli to which it was paying attention at that particular moment (totally identical in terms of physical characteristics to those disregarded). This implied that it was possible to study mental processes by observing their neurophysiologic manifestations.

To study language, Marta Kutas developed two different experimental paradigms. In the first, rapid serial visual presentation (RSVP), single words are consecutively presented in the center of a screen [7] in order to simulate the process involved in the spontaneous reading of a sentence and to monitor the time course of semantic and syntactic comprehension processes, while avoiding the horizontal ocular movements that normally go along with text reading. In fact, any ERP recording paradigm assumes complete gaze fixity, thereby avoiding EEG contamination by electromyographic signals.

The second, quite popular paradigm is called the "terminal word" [8] and it is based on the presentation of a semantic or syntactic context of variable nature and complexity that is followed by a given terminal word, to which the evoked potential is time-locked and which can be more or less congruent with the context or respectful of various word concatenation rules of a given language. An example of this paradigm is shown by the sentences in Fig. 4.1. In the following paragraphs, the various stages of linguistic information processes, ranging from orthographic to syntactic analysis, are discussed in a greater detail as are more complex ERP components not illustrated in Fig. 4.1 (such as ELAN, LAN, and SPS, which are defined and discussed in Par. 4.8).

4.3 Orthographic Analysis

A widely debated question in the recent neuroimaging literature [9-12] concerns the existence of a cerebral area specialized in the visual analysis of orthographic stimuli and words, called the visual word form area (VWFA), which lies in the left inferotemporal cortex and, more precisely, in the fusiform gyrus (Fig. 4.3). Neurofunctional studies have shown that this region responds with higher activation to linguistic stimuli (alphabetic strings) than to non-linguistic stimuli (such as checkerboards), and to real characters to a greater extent than to false characters or symbolic or iconic strings (Fig. 4.3) [9, 11, 13-17].

It also seems that the VWFA has a certain degree of sublexical sensitivity to the orthographic regularities with which letters form words. Indeed, fMRI data [13] have

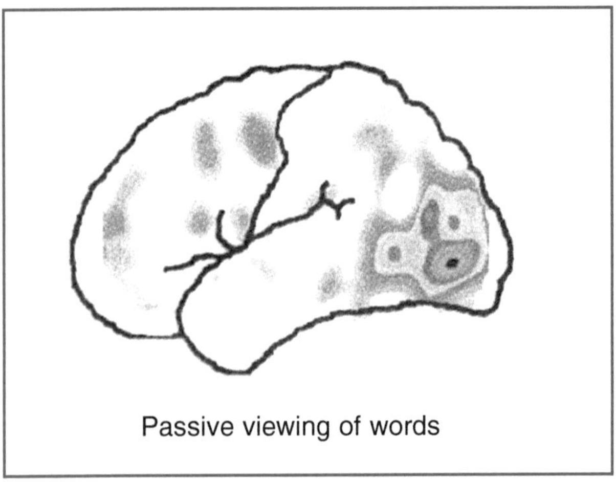

Fig. 4.3 The passive visualization of words (with respect to non-linguistic stimuli) activates the left occipito-temporal cortex

evidenced that this region is more active in response to well-structured letter strings (legal pseudo-words) than to those which are ill-structured (i.e., illegal strings). The data also suggest that the VWFA distinguishes meaningful legal strings (words) from legal pseudo-words [10, 18].

It can be hypothesized that functionally different levels of processing take place in the same area. Thus, there may be a first level of processing in which some micropopulations of neurons recognize alphabetic letters, discriminating them from unknown symbolic systems (in this case letters are treated as familiar visual objects), followed by a more complex level in which VWFA neurons, with a receptive field larger than neurons of the first level, discriminate pseudo-words from words (in this case, familiar visual objects are over-learned letter strings, i.e., words).

ERPs represent a quite useful tool for investigating reading mechanisms in that they provide several indices of what is occurring in the brain, millisecond by millisecond, starting from stimulus onset: from the analysis of sensory visual characteristics (curved or straight lines, angles, circles), to orthographic analysis (letter recognition), to the analysis of complex patterns (words) and their orthographic aspect (which, for example, greatly differs for the German, English, or Finnish languages) and their meaning.

Numerous ERP and MEG studies have provided clear evidence that the occipito-temporal N1 ERP response (with a mean latency of 150–200 ms) specifically reflects stimulus orthographic analysis [15, 19-24]. For example, Helenius and coworkers [20] recorded MEG signals in dyslexic and control adult individuals engaged in silent reading or the visualization of symbolic strings either clearly visible or degraded with Gaussian noise. The results showed that while the first sensory response (at about 100 ms of latency), originating in the extrastriate cortex and associated with variations in luminance contrast, did not differ in amplitude in dyslexics *vs* normal readers, the first component sensitive to orthographic factors, a N150 that was generated in the left inferior occipito-temporal cortex, and thus probably in the VWFA (see Fig. 4.4), was not observable in dyslexic individuals. Similarly, fMRI and MEG

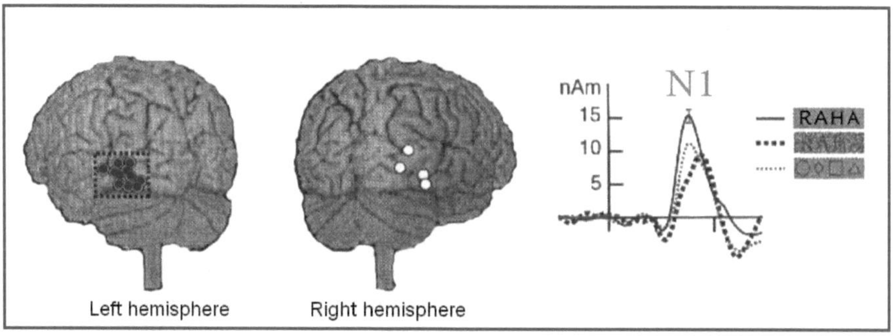

Fig. 4.4 (Electromagnetic) N170 (mN170) in response to letter strings, degraded letters, and geometric symbols in non-dyslexic adult individuals. Maps show the anatomical localization and strong hemispheric asymmetry in visual word form area (VWFA) activation. (Modified from Helenius et al. [20], with permission of the authors and Oxford University Press)

4

studies in adult individuals with developmental dyslexia [24] or in children with reading disorders [25] have shown insufficient/atypical activation of left posterior regions during reading.

In a recent study [26], we compared ERPs evoked by words and pseudo-words in their canonical orientation with those elicited by words and pseudo-words specularly rotated. The aim was to assess whether the inversion of words deprived them of their linguistic properties, thus making them non-linguistic stimuli. An EEG was recorded from 128 channels and slightly fewer than 1300 stimuli were presented, half of which were words and the other half pseudo-words. The task consisted of detecting a given letter (which might be included, or not, in the stimuli) that was announced by the experimenter at the beginning of each trial. In order to identify the temporal latency of alphabetic letter processing and recognition, ERPs evoked by target and non-target stimuli were compared. The lateral-occipital N170 ERP component was found to be involved in this process, as it was of larger amplitude for targets than for non-targets. A LORETA analysis, which identifies the anatomical sources of bioelectrical signals, carried out on the ERP difference wave, obtained by subtracting the N1 to target letters from that to non-targets, showed a strong focus of activation in the left fusiform gyrus (BA 37; x = -29.5, y = -43, z = -14.3), probably corresponding to the VWFA. The contrast between ERPs elicited by mirror *vs* standard stimuli revealed instead a non-linguistic effect (at the occipito-temporal N1 level too). LORETA analysis, conducted on the difference wave obtained by subtracting the N1 to standard stimuli from the N1 to mirror words, identified a source of activation elicited by word inversion in the right medial occipital gyrus (BA 19; x = 37.7, y = -68.1; z = -4.6). This finding evidenced the activation of a non-linguistic visual area for processing strings of different familiarity, and of a VWFA dedicated to the actual orthographic analysis (letter recognition). This finding suggests some caveats in the excessive and mindless use of the object inversion paradigm in neuroimaging research (for studying face, house, and object processing) to investigate the existence of regions responding to specific semantic and functional categories.

4.4
Phonologic/Phonetic Analysis

It is widely known that the second stage of analysis in the reading process is represented by the conversion of the visual form into the phonologic one, also referred to as grapheme-to-phoneme conversion. A recent event-related fMRI study [27] investigated this mechanism in word reading, finding a larger activation of left inferior frontal gyrus for pseudo-word reading as well as a greater bilateral activation of occipito-temporal areas and of the left posterior medial temporal gyrus during the reading of words and letter strings, at about 170–230 ms of latency. Other studies are in agreement with a role for the left inferior frontal cortex in pseudo-word reading [28]. This region may belong to the above-mentioned phonologic route, postulated to be involved in the assembling of phonologic segments (*assembled phonology*) during reading. The magnetic source imaging study by Simos and coworkers [29] confirmed the existence of two different mechanisms involved in phonologic processing during word visual recognition: one supporting assembled phonology for reading legal but inexistent strings, and depending on the activation of the superior segment of the superior temporal gyrus (STG), and another supporting phonology addressed to real word reading, dependent on the left posterior medial temporal gyrus. These recent neuroimaging studies are consistent with what is predicted by the so-called computational two-way reading model (see [1] for a review), which assumes one routine addressing the pronunciation of words recognized by the reader (the lexical-semantic route) and another responsible for assembling the pronunciation of inexistent strings, based on a grapheme/phoneme correspondence (spelling-sound), i.e., the phonologic route.

Despite this approach to understanding the neuroanatomical basis of grapheme-to-phoneme conversion processes, only cerebral electromagnetic signals, and especially ERPs, can precisely determine the temporal course of analysis of the phonetic/phonologic aspects of reading. And indeed, ERPs have been used in several studies aimed at investigating the time course of the phonetic/phonologic processing stage for written words, especially by means of rhyme judgement paradigms [19, 30, 31], in which subjects are asked to evaluate whether a series of words rhyme with each other (for example, if PLATE rhymes with EIGHT or with VIOLET). Typically, items incongruent from the phonologic point of view, i.e., not rhyming, elicit a negative response of *mismatch*, whose latency indicates the temporal stage of phonologic processing (around 250 ms).

In a study by Bentin and co-workers [19], ERPs elicited by words and pseudowords that rhymed with a given French word were compared with ERPs elicited by non-rhyming words. The results showed the presence of a negative component at around 320 ms of post-stimulus latency, reaching a maximum amplitude over the left medial temporal region in response to non-rhyming items. Functional neuroimaging studies [32] have shown that the dorsal areas surrounding the Heschl gyrus, bilaterally, and in particular the planum temporalis and the dorsolateral STG, are activated to a greater degree during the processing of frequency-modulated tones rather than noise, suggesting their role in the processing of temporally coded simple auditory information. By contrast, regions centered in the superior temporal sulcus are more active, bilaterally, during listening to linguistic stimuli (both words and pseudowords, or *inverted speech*) rather than tones, suggesting their role in pre-phonetic acoustic processing. Lastly, ventral temporal and temporo-parietal areas are more active during the processing of words and non-words, suggesting their role in accessing the phonologic and semantic properties of words.

Therefore, while neuroimaging studies indicate the possible neuroanatomical substrates of word phonologic analysis mechanisms, electromagnetic studies (ERP and MEG) provide the temporal progression of processing stages (250–350 ms), as shown in Proverbio's and Zani's study [31] and illustrated in Figure 4.5. This figure shows the *phonologic mismatch negativity* (pMMN) in response to incongruent trigrams with respect to given words held in memory for a few seconds. Volunteers were asked to access the phonologic form of words described by means of a unique

4

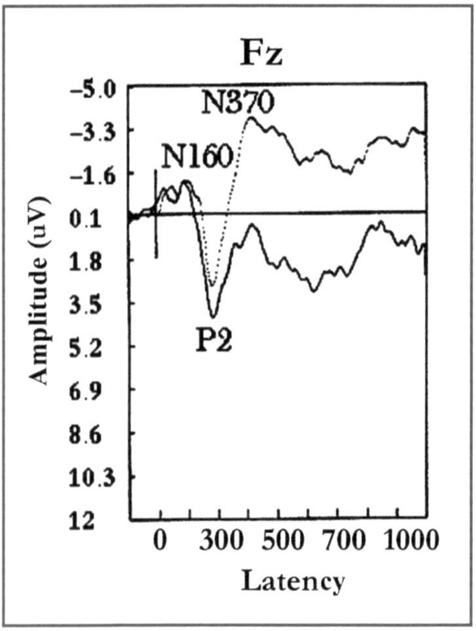

Fig. 4.5 Phonologic mismatch negativity (pMMN) in response to syllables phonologically incongruent with the phonologic form of the words retrieved and held in memory by the observer. Note the early onset of negativity, around 200 ms of post-stimulus latency. (From Proverbio and Zani [33], Fig. 2, copyright 2003, with the permission of Elsevier)

definition. For example: "collects and sells old furniture:" ANTIQUARIAN, or "boundary between two countries:" BORDER. Subsequently, volunteers were required to establish whether or not a trigram, successively presented after a given interval, was part of the word thought, by pressing one of two buttons indicating an affirmative or negative answer. In the above example, QUA is present in ANTIQUARIAN (key: YES), whereas LEN is not (key: NO). Under these experimental conditions, the phonologic representation of words was not provided according to a given sensory modality (visual if written or auditory if spoken) but to a mental abstract code.

In that study, pMMN provided the mean latency of occurrence of language phonologic analysis processes (about 250–350 ms); however, an earlier index of grapheme-to-phoneme conversion activity for written words was found, in particular for trigram processing. A visual MMN was observed in this study over the extra-striate visual cortex–and, more precociously, over the left hemisphere–during a comparison of phonologically incongruent syllables, hence suggesting an access to syllable and word phonologic properties and the onset of grapheme-to-phoneme conversion process at about 175 ms post-stimulus.

Another, recent ERP study further investigated grapheme-to-phoneme conversion mechanisms [23], highlighting the time course of mechanisms supporting the extraction of phonetic information during reading. The experimental paradigm was the following: more than one thousand Italian words, pseudo-words, and letter strings were presented to Italian university students whose task was to establish whether a given phone was present in a visually provided word. A phone corresponds to the acoustic/phonetic implementation of a given phoneme (and therefore grapheme) and is only accessible if the pronunciation rules are precisely known and pronunciation ambiguities are not possible, not even for pseudo-words or letter strings. For example, in Italian, the C grapheme is definitely pronounced [tʃ], both in the word CIELO (sky) and in the pseudo-word CERTUBIOLA or in the string MLHGWTOCIV, as every Italian speaker who masters grapheme-to-phoneme conversion rules for the Italian language knows very well (in addition, Italian is a transparent language; see Table 4.1 for a list of phones used as targets as well as those used as distracters in order to make the task more difficult). ERPs to all stimulus categories (according to whether or not they contained target phones) were then recorded.

Table 4.1 List of target phones to be responded to in a given trial, along with distracter phones included in half of the non-target items. Distracters might have an orthographic or a phonetic similarity with the targets. (From Proverbio et al. [23], with the permission of MIT Press)

Target			Non-target
Phone	Graphemee	Example	Distractors
[k]	c	cuore	[tʃ], [ʃ] bacio, sciata,
[tʃ]	c	cielo	[k], [ʃ], [kw] occhio, fascio,
[ʃ]	sc	pesce	[s], [k], [tʃ], [kw] secchio, carta falce, eloquio
[z]	s	isola	[s], [ts], [ʃ], [dz] sodio, sensazione, uscita, zia
[s]	s	pasta	[z], [ts], [ʃ], causa, fazione,biscia
[ts]	z	pizza	[s], [dz], [z] bistecca, manzo, revisore
[dz]	z	zaino	[ts], [s], [z] polizia, sigaretta, riserva
[g]	g	gatto	[ɲ], [dʒ], [ʎ] sogno, gesto, sveglia
[dʒ]	g	gente	[ʎ], [ɲ], [g] voglia, prugna, ghiaccio
[ʎ]	gl	aglio	[l], [g], [dʒ], [ɲ] palio, lingua, gioco, montagna
[ɲ]	gn	pugno	[n], [g], [dʒ], [ʎ] banana, ghiacciolo, formaggio, sbaglio
[n]	n	brina	[ɲ], [ʎ] ragno, boscaglia

Among the most interesting data was the anterior/posterior functional anatomical dissociation observed for a negative component around 250–350 ms, which was of larger amplitude over frontal and left prefrontal regions during phonemic processing of well-formed letter strings (pseudo-words) or ill-formed strings, but reached its maximum amplitude over left occipito-temporal regions during phonemic analysis of high or low frequency words [23]. This finding supports the possible existence of two functionally distinct circuits (one visual and the other phonologic) for grapheme-to-phoneme conversion. It also indicates the time course of such processes, which partially occur in parallel with the completion of word visual recognition from the VWFA and the beginning of access to the lexical system indexed by the subsequent N400 component, with a latency ranging from 200 to 600 ms. Quick access to word phonologic/phonetic representation allows us to read at high speed, as many as five or six words per second, even complicated and unknown text passages. Reading ability obviously develops with exercise and improves from infancy to adulthood. Some fMRI studies (e.g., [34]) have demonstrated that fast and accurate access to phonologic representation is significantly improved in adult *vs* prepubertal (until 14 years) individuals and that during adolescence both a refinement of reading abilities and the further consolidation of automatisms in reading processes occur. In particular, Booth and co-workers [35] showed modifications related to brain development and age in the activation of linguistic left cortical areas during reading, especially involving the inferior frontal area, STG, and angular gyrus. During intermodal auditory/visual tasks (for example, visual rhyme tasks such as: does SOAP [səʊp] rhyme with HOPE [həʊp]?), specific activation of the angular gyrus (BA39), involved in mapping of the correspondence between orthographic and phonologic word representations, was recorded both in prepubertal individuals and in adults. What was most interesting is that, in adults, automatic activation of the angular gyrus was observed also during orthographic tasks not requiring grapheme-to-phoneme conversion, as in the task: does VOTE [vəʊt] rhyme with NOTE [nəʊt]? This type of automatic activation was not observable in prepubertal individuals, probably because of maturational differences in synaptogenesis, glucose metabolism, myelinization, and cortical white matter development, occurring between 10 and 20 ms and especially in prefrontal areas. Thus, the findings of Booth and co-workers [35] essentially identified, in the angular and supramarginal gyri, a region specialized in the orthographic/phonologic *mapping* of linguistic information. In addition, during the transition from puberty to adulthood, these same findings point to an improvement in nervous signal transmission and the fast interconnection of heteromodal regions in reading.

4.5
Grapheme-to-phoneme Conversion in Reading Deficits (Dyslexia)

Reading disabilities, in the sense of deficits in the fast retrieval of grapheme/phoneme correspondences–and therefore the graphemic form in dictation (i.e., how to write something that has been heard) and the phonetic form in reading (i.e., how to pronounce something that has been read)–are found in some dyslexic children and are mostly of the phonologic type. As described in Par. 4.2, certain subjects (i.e., those with surface dyslexia) may exhibit an insufficient/atypical activation of the VWFA [20], which, as discussed in the study of Proverbio et al., is partly involved in graphemic/phonologic analysis [33]. However, most of the theories on the neurobiological bases of phonologic dyslexia refer to three main hypotheses. These are discussed below in the context of electrophysiological data (except for the so-called magnocellular hypothesis, which assumes an involvement of ocular-movement-related structures and of the cerebellum, which will not be treated here).

The first hypothesis is that dyslexics suffer from a deficit in their ability to discriminate temporally complex acoustic information; however, it should be immediately clarified that the contrary has been widely shown by means of non-linguistic-type stimuli. The second hypothesis is that they suffer from a deficit in the ability to discriminate among formant transition times (especially shortest *vs* longer times). The third hypothesis, which, as we will see later, is supported by electromagnetic and neuroimaging data, is that dyslexics suffer from a deficit in phonetic discrimination due to the *allophonic perception* of linguistic stimuli. Allophonic perception is very sensitive to subtle physical variations in sound stimulation in terms of formant transition times, but it is accompanied by an unstable grapheme/phoneme correspondence (confusions in global shape categorization of the signal spectrum).

The hypothesis of a deficit in temporal discrimination was disconfirmed in recent studies such as those by Studdert-Kennedy and Nittrouer, both of which showed that deficits in phonetic awareness do not depend on problems in the auditory processing of temporally complex or fast information. Indeed, 2nd-grade schoolchildren with troubles in distinguishing /ba/-/da/ syllables do just as well as same-age normal readers in tasks involving syllable discriminations with a similar degree of temporal complexity in formant transition times but phonetically more distinctive for place and type of articulation (such as (/ba/-/sa/, or /fa/-/da/); they are equally good in tasks requiring a sensitivity to short transition signals of synthetic speech, or in discriminating non-linguistic sound waves similar in the second and third formant of syllables /ba/ and /da/. Thus, dyslexic children, rather than having troubles in detecting rapid changes in the acoustic information spectrum [36], might suffer from the perceptual confounding of phonetically similar phonemes. This hypothesis is supported by electrophysiological studies making use of synthetic speech. A specific paradigm that has highlighted a deficit of a phonologic rather than of an acoustic/phonetic nature in dyslexic children is the implicit phonologic priming, which can occur in lexical decision tasks (deciding whether a stimulus is a word or a non-word) by previously presenting a prime word that can be (or not) phonologically related to the following target stimuli. For example, MORNING acts as a phonologic prime (facilitating agent) for the pseudo-word CORNING but not for the pseudo-word LEBANTI. A lack or reduction in the pMMN for phonologically unrelated *vs* related items is typically found in the presence of a deficit (Fig. 4.6).

As previously stated, a phonologic deficit is not associated with a lack of acoustic/phonetic sensitivity but, instead, with an extreme sensitivity to temporal rather than spatial (spectrum) indices. It has been demonstrated [37] that dyslexics

4

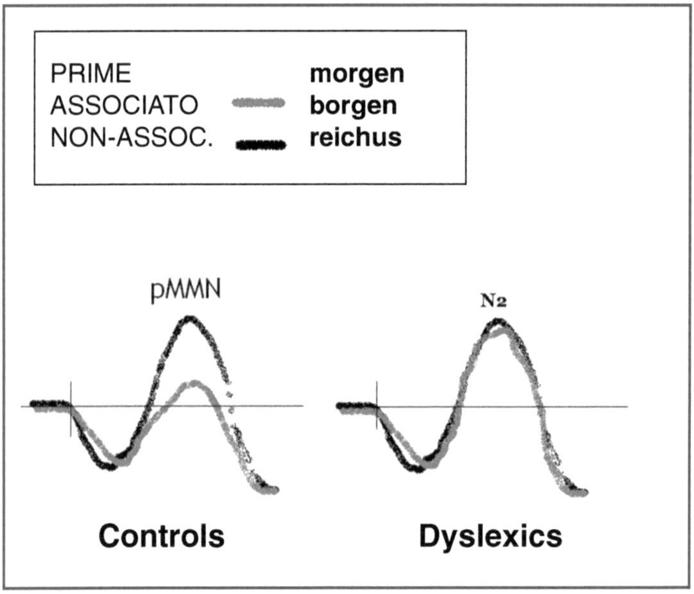

Fig. 4.6 ERP waveforms recorded in dyslexic individuals and controls in response to pseudo-words phonologically related or unrelated to a previous word (prime). The lack of discriminative response between the two stimulus types at the temporo-parietal N2 level reflects a specific deficit in phonologic processing

perform better than controls in intra-category syllable discrimination tasks with synthetic syllable obtained by imperceptibly modifying two clearly discriminable syllables, such as /da/ and /ta/, along a continuum of intermediate stimuli. By contrast, dyslexic individuals perform worst in syllable discrimination tasks when phonemes are categorically different (e.g., /da/ *vs* /ta/). Figure 4.7 shows the data of a phonemic categorization study performed with synthetic speech and evidences an incompetence in 10-year-old children with respect to establishing a correspondence between phonologic input and phonemic representation, similar to that of non-dyslexic 6-year-old children not yet able to read or at least extremely insecure about precise grapheme/phoneme mapping.

This marked sensitivity to differences in the continuum of auditory stimulation is, as noted above, referred to as allophonic perception, in contrast to categorical perception. The demonstration that dyslexics are more sensitive to phonetic differences derives from ERP studies making use of the MMN paradigm, developed by Finnish scientist Risto Näätänen [38, 39]. This paradigm is based on the acoustic presentation of a repetitive series of homogeneous stimuli followed by a stimulus deviant for a single physical characteristic (for example, duration, intensity, frequency, or spectrum). A comparison between ERPs elicited by standard *vs* deviant stimuli showed a negativity whose latency (150–300 ms) and localization indicated the neural mechanisms

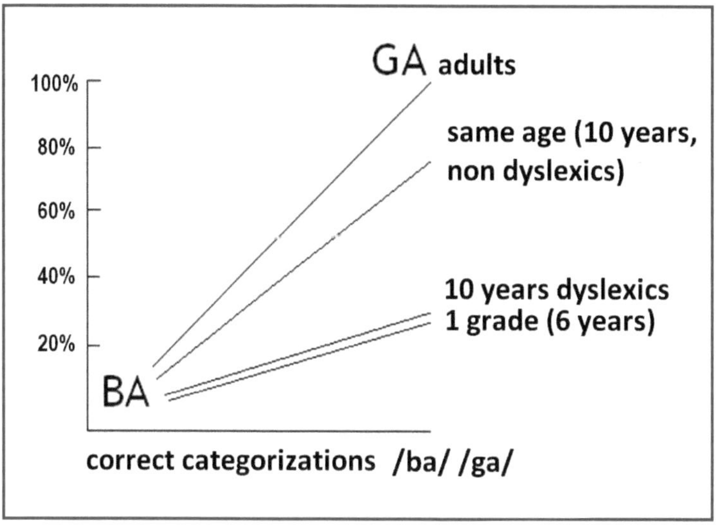

Fig. 4.7 Comparison among performances attained in a synthetic phoneme categorization task by groups of speakers of different ages and phonological competence. The performances of 10-year-old dyslexic children were similar to those of first-grade schoolchildren

processing the deviant sensory characteristics. In tasks in which a series of words clearly pronounced without skating over some letters (e.g., ALREADY) were compared with words pronounced according to some assimilation rules (e.g., A(L)READY), dyslexic patients seem to show a larger MMN, both earlier (340 ms) and later (520 ms), than determined in controls. Essentially, controls compensate for differences in phonetic information in order to come to similar final categorization, whereas dyslexic individuals are more sensitive to phonetic differences in stimulation, thus giving rise to greater negativity from acoustic/phonetic mismatch in response to words such as A(L)READY (assimilated) *vs* ALREADY (clearly pronounced).

Further proof of the greater sensitivity of dyslexics to deviant stimuli comes from an electrophysiological study by Pavo Leppänen et al. [40], who compared the responses evoked by standard or deviant words in terms of a vowel or consonant duration. For example, the word /**tu**li/ (fire) was contrasted with the deviant word /**tuu**li/ (wind), differing just for the vowel duration /u/, whereas the standard segment /a**t**a/ was contrasted with the longer version /a**tt**a/. This authoritative longitudinal study was carried out on a population of 100 6-month-old newborns belonging to families without reading deficits, and therefore genetically not prone to dyslexia (controls), and another 100 children belonging to families in which at least one member had a reading deficit. The results showed a much larger MMN, especially in the late phase (600 ms) in response to deviant stimuli in at-risk newborns. The monitoring of at-risk individuals in their adult age then showed that a certain percentage of them actually developed a reading deficit. MMN recorded in dyslexics individuals (that is poor readers, of the at-risk group) in response to stimuli, such as /ka/ standard *vs* /kaa/ deviant, was of significant amplitude, but predominantly observable over right hemispheric regions. MMN recorded in individuals originally at risk but who never developed reading problems (that is, good readers, at-risk group) showed good amplitude over both the right and left hemispheric regions. Finally, MMN recorded in good readers (not at risk) showed a single MMN over left hemispheric regions. Therefore, it seems that a right MMN was somewhat predictive of a predisposition to confusion in phonemic categorization. This finding might be related to evidence that people with less-pronounced manual preferences have a greater probability of suffering from dyslexia than strongly right-handed individuals. Electrophysiological studies have shown a clear improvement in reading ability in 5-year-old children with a poor sound/letter association ability (and belonging to genetically at-risk families, that is, with at least one dyslexic family member) after specific, intensive training. ERP data provided evidence of a significant correlation between improvement in the ability to correctly read letters and the appearance of an early MMN over the left temporo-parietal regions in response to the standard/deviant contrast for /ba/ /ga/ /da/ phoneme types.

This type of training, devised to capture the attention of 5- to 6-year-old children, consisted of a video-game called the "graphogame," in which the child listens to sounds presented individually via headphones while he/she watches a PC screen. In order to win the game, the child has to readily catch the orthographic version within the time corresponding to the vocal sound heard (represented as a vertically falling letter) before it lands, by moving a cursor (a friendly U-shape little polyp) with open tentacles. Different letters land simultaneously such that it is necessary to be very quick in identifying and catching the right one to win the various levels of the videogame. Graphogame and its effects on cortical plasticity and learning have been of interest since 2005, in the context of the VI European Union Framework Program aimed at studying reading problems in English-, Finnish-, Dutch-, or German-speaking children, through a project entitled "Training grapheme-phoneme correlations with a child-friendly computer game in preschool children with familial risk of dyslexia."

In summary, learning to read consists in establishing a stable and reliable grapheme/phoneme correspondence. This, as previously noted, is a constantly improving process that continues to improves after puberty, in part due to the crucial role of the angular and supramarginal gyri, whereas a slight weakness in the phonologic coding of phonetic inputs (phonemic categorization) predisposes a child to dyslexia.

4.6 Lexical Analysis

After accessing phonologic word properties, the brain is able to extract its semantic/lexical properties at around 300–400 ms of post-stimulus latency. In 1980, by means of the terminal word paradigm [8], it was possible to determine the existence of a negative ERP component of about 400 ms of latency (named N400), which emerged in response to words semantically incongruent with the context but orthographically and phonologically correct. The amplitude of this component is generally greater over the right centro-parietal area, although this does not necessarily correspond to the anatomical localization of semantic functions. For example, intracranial recording studies have shown N400 generators near the collateral sulcus and the anterior fusiform gyrus. In her original 1980 paper, Kutas used the terminal word paradigm to describe the functional properties of N400, distinguishing between the concepts of semantic incongruence and subjective expectation of sentence termination. Thus, Kutas postulated a *contextual constraint* induced by the semantic meaning of the sentence, which in itself would not be sufficient to explain the increased N400. To explain this with an example, the incongruence between the sentence "He/she put sugar and lemon in his/her TEA" and "He/she put sugar and lemon in his/her BOOT" produces a N400 of noticeable magnitude in response to the word BOOT because of the semantic incongruence of this terminal word within the context of the type of warm drink. Compared to the response induced by the sentence "He/she put sugar and lemon in his/her COFFEE", a N400 of lesser amplitude in response to the terminal word COFFEE than to the word BOOT can be appreciated because the former word is semantically more related to the word TEA than the latter. This finding reflects the effect of the *contextual constraint.*

Kutas also introduced the *cloze probability* or *closure probability* factor, meant as the probability that a group of speakers might complete a certain sentence with a specific terminal word whose effects do not completely correspond to those of the contextual constraint. For instance, the sentence "He/she sent his/her letter without a STAMP" is completed in a uniform and predictable way by all speakers, because it has a high cloze probability. Conversely, the sentence "There was not anything wrong with the FREEZER" has a low cloze probability since, from a statistical point of view, not many speakers would complete this sentence the same way. Indeed, ERPs elicited by the words STAMP and FREEZER in the aforementioned sentences show much different deflections (P300 and N400, respectively) since the word FREEZER surprises the reader as much as would any other word representing another object whose mechanism might have a glitch, as it is also certainly semantically congruent but nonetheless unexpected.

The N400 is a hallmark of the mechanisms of semantic integration, and, as such, sensitive to the difficulty with which the reader/listener integrates the ongoing sensory input with the previous context, based on the individual expectations.

Although the maximum response peak to incompatible, unexpected, or low cloze probability words is reached around 400 ms, earlier ERP responses have also been reported as being sensitive to some lexical properties of words, such as their frequency of use. King and Kutas [41] described an anterior negative component, the *lexical processing negativity* (LPN), with a latency of about 280–340 ms, which was shown to be very sensitive to the frequency of word occurrence. This component, also recorded in the above-mentioned study by Proverbio and co-workers [23], is based on a phonetic decision task, as illustrated in Fig. 4.8, which shows the LPN recorded in response to various stimulus categories of different familiarity to the readers (strings,

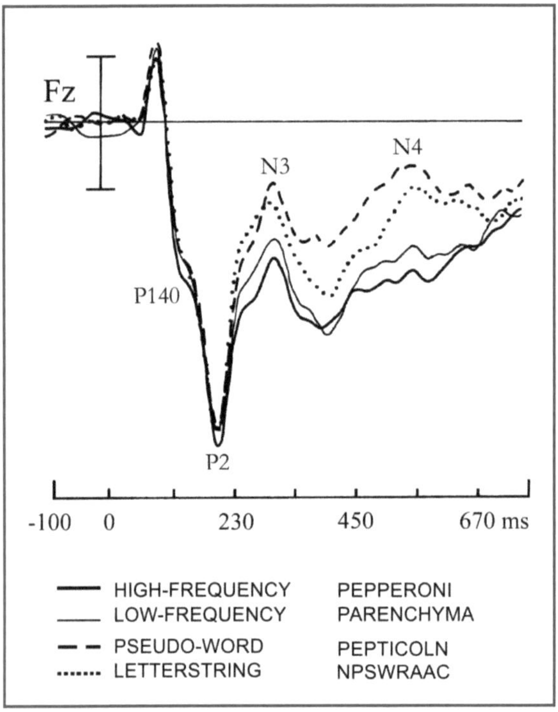

Fig. 4.8 ERP waveforms recorded in response to words, pseudo-words, and letter strings during a phonetic decision task (e.g., "Is phone /k/ present in oranges?"). (Modified from Proverbio et al. [23], with the permission of MIT Press)

pseudo-words, and words of high and low frequency of use). Noteworthy is how familiarity affected the magnitude of the N3 and N4 subcomponents of the LPN, even if the phonetic task did not require any access to the lexical level of stimulus information. Lexical effects were already evident at 250 ms of post-stimulus latency over the anterior brain regions, and still earlier (around 150 ms) over the parietal cortex, in the form of a modulation of the amplitude of the P150. Consistently, in another ERP study, Schendan and colleagues [42] described a P150 central-parietal component of maximum amplitude in response to letter strings and pseudo-letters, intermediate magnitude in response to icon strings, and low amplitude in response to objects and pseudo-objects. Based on these findings, the authors concluded that the P150 might well be the scalp reflection of an intracranial source localized in the fusiform gyrus.

In our study [23], the earliest effects of the lexical distinction (i.e., word *vs* pseudo-word) were observed at about 200 ms post-stimulus. It would seem, then, that neural mechanisms of access to the lexical features of linguistic stimuli activate in parallel with the extraction of their orthographic and phonologic properties. Some studies also demonstrated a sensitivity to the lexical properties of the left-sided central-parietal region at latencies still earlier than 150 ms in response to short, familiar words [43, 44].

4.7 Pragmatic Analysis

Just as the P300 represents an index at the scalp of the neural mechanisms of *contextual updating*, in other words, the updating of personal knowledge as a consequence of comparing the ongoing stimulus input with the information retained in long-term memory stores [45, 46], conversely, an increased N400 represents a difficulty in the attempt to integrate ongoing input with previous knowledge of a semantic or procedural nature (as with sign language), world knowledge of a pragmatic nature, and social knowledge (scenarios, conventions or customs, and behavior appropriateness). Some examples, discussed individually, are provided in the following.

First, let us take the classical example of a violation of the local meaning or semantic constraint such as the one provided by the sentence "Jane told her brother that he was very...," followed by three possible terminal words:

A. FAST Congruent;
B. SLOW Congruent;
C. RAINY Incongruent.

As extensively dealt with in the previous paragraph, case C gives rise to a N400 (depicted in Fig. 4.9, case 1) since "rainy-ness" is not a possible property of a person, which therefore makes it hard to integrate the meaning of the terminal word with the conceptual representation elicited by the aforementioned sentence. Since this incongruence is verifiable per se, independently of the context or the specific speakers, it is defined as a violation of the semantic constraint (which is to be distinguished by the cloze probability).

However, Hagoorth and co-workers (e.g., [47]) discovered that the N400 is also sensitive to violation of the sentence meaning, mediated by the context or by social knowledge. Let us consider, for instance, the context: "At 7:00 a.m., Jane's brother had already taken a shower and had dressed too," followed by the sentence "Jane told her brother that he was incredibly...," completed by the terminal words:

A. FAST Congruent;
B. SLOW Incongruent.

Case B therefore also gives rise to a N400 (depicted in Fig. 4.9, case 2) since the conceptual representation of a fast and early-rising brother elicited by the quoted sentence is in striking contrast with the way his sister defines him. The semantic incongruence can be extended to implicit or pragmatic knowledge, such as social knowledge. Let us consider, for instance, a sentence as "On Sundays, I usually go to the park with..." pronounced by the voice of: (1) a child and (2) an adult man, and followed by two possible terminal words:

A. MY DADDY;
B. MY WIFE.

Instances 1B and 2A elicit a wide N400 deflection (Fig. 4.9, case 3) in the absence of any violation of the local and/or contextual semantic meaning, thus indexing a pure violation of pragmatic and/or social knowledge.

Another study by Hagoort and colleagues [48] provided a very interesting paral-

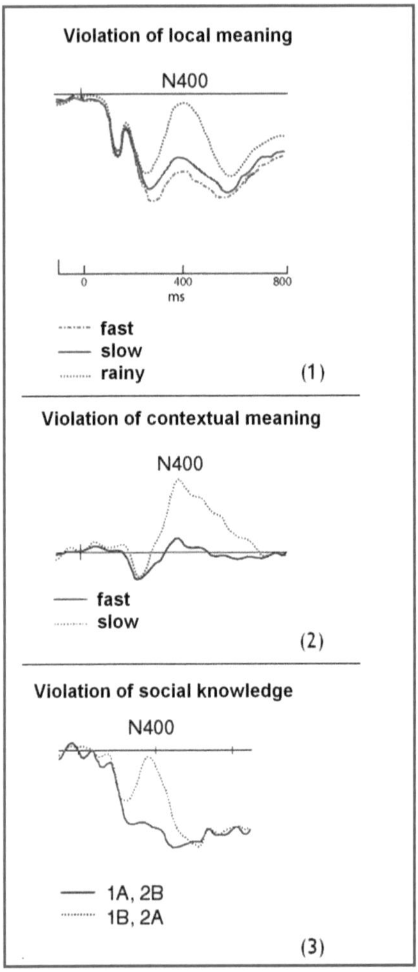

Fig. 4.9 ERP recorded in response to terminal words completing a previous context (see the text for specific sentences) determining a violation of local meaning (case 1), contextual meaning (case 2), or pragmatic knowledge (case 3). *Dotter line*, incongruent word, *solid line*, congruent word. (Modified from studies of Hagoort et al. [47,48], with permission of the authors)

lelism between violation of the semantic constraint and violation of world knowledge. A typical example of *world knowledge* (as defined by the cognitive psychologist Donald Norman) could be the direction that doors open (almost always inwards, but outwards in case of anti-panic doors), a knowledge that is implicitly learned by means of repeated experience with the external world. Hagoort comparatively presented three types of sentences:

A. Dutch trains are yellow and very crowded.
B. Dutch trains are white and very crowded.
C. Dutch trains are sour and very crowded.

Sentences B (i.e., a violation of world knowledge) and C (i.e., a semantic violation) elicited N400s of similar amplitudes and topographic distributions in Dutch participants, although these violations were extremely different in type. Everyone knows that a train cannot be acidic (semantic knowledge). Similarly, a Dutch person who has traveled by subway and/or railway would implicitly, and robustly, be aware of the fact that the trains of his/her town and/or country are not white.

The difficulty in integrating the information provided by sentences B and C with pre-existing knowledge thus induces mental processes observable about 400 ms after the target word, the neurophysiological counterpart of which is represented by the N400, and whose intracranial source in both cases has been localized, by means of fMRI, to the left inferior frontal gyrus (BA45) [48].

4.8 First- and Second-level Syntactic Analysis

The syntactic analysis of a sentence, that is analysis of the relationships across the various parts of the discourse, in both written and oral forms, consists of diverse, more or less complex processing levels. These occur in parallel with the other types of linguistic signal processing, while recognition outputs are progressively derived from orthographic, phonologic, and semantic analyses. The initial stages are more automatic and less affected by expectancies and cognitive representations. Indeed, according to Noam Chomsky, a certain syntactic skill or *universal grammar* (the ability to understand and then generate a discourse based on specific syntactic rules) is innate and inherent to the biological architecture of *Homo sapiens*. ERP studies have allowed the disentangling of three different types of partially consecutive analyses, whose neurophysiological indexes over the scalp consist of the ELAN, LAN, and P600 or SPS, which will be dealt with below.

Early left anterior negativity (ELAN) can be recorded around a latency range between 100 and 300 ms over the anterior regions of the brain [49]. It reflects the mechanisms of syntactic attribution and integration of a sentence and is very sensitive to the categories of the various parts of the discourse. Typically, a sentence such as "Home the girl came back" elicits an early ELAN due to a form of syntactic violation, since the various parts of the discourse do not hold the positions that they should (i.e., article, nominal syntagm, verbal syntagm, adverbial syntagm). Thus, ELAN would reflect a first-level parsing, driven by the rules for the construction of a sentence and by primary (partially innate) syntactic processes.

Late anterior negativity (LAN) [50, 51] is also an anterior negativity linked to syntactic violations, but it is recorded at a later latency (i.e., 300–500 ms) and sensitive to more complex morphological-syntactic linguistic factors, such as subject/verb and verb/article agreements, declensions, and conjugations. A sentence that would usually elicit a remarkably large LAN might be "The boys will has gone."

A third and more complex level of syntactic analysis is represented by a positive component called the *syntactic positive shift* (SPS), or P600, because of its occurrence around 600 ms post-stimulus [52, 53]. Following the P300, this component rises only after the acquisition of a certain awareness of the meaning of a sentence. This late positivity reflects relatively controlled linguistic processes, more sensitive to inflexional information, and is somehow linked to secondary syntactic processes, such as the re-analysis of complex and incongruent sentences or the suppression of incorrect representations of those sentences due to certain difficulties in syntactic integration. Presumably, to understand these sentences, one would have had to invoke secondary syntactic processes, whose ERP surface reflection would consist of a P600. Let us consider the sentence "The child could not keep a thing in...," and let us assume that there is a certain time span during which the reader, or the listener, has enough time to build up a mental representation of the sentence meaning, and thus a specific expectation of the terminal word. Quite off the point, the presentation of a conclusion such as "his torn pants pockets" instead of "his head" induces re-analysis processes of the meaning of the sentence, and in particular of the word "keep," which had been almost certainly interpreted as "to remember." The unexpected conclusion changes the meaning of the verb "keep" from its semantic acceptation of "remembering" into its acceptation of "holding," thus compelling the reader/listener to a re-analysis of the sentence, indexed at the surface by the SPS.

Furthermore, Kutas and colleagues described other interesting linguistic components [54], such as the left anterior negativity related to the syntactic complexity of the sentence, which are rather specific and reflect the involvement of the left frontal cortex (e. g., Broca's area) in syntactic analysis. The same authors carried out a study comparing syntactically complex sentences, such as those with object-relative clauses, with those consisting of other, globally identical subject-relative clauses. For instance, the sentence "The reporter who the senator harshly attacked admitted the error" (an object-relative clause) was compared to the sentence "The reporter who harshly attacked the senator admitted the error" (a subject-relative clause). The ERPs were recorded off-line in a group of participants divided in two sub-groups as a function of their comprehension level of the sentences. The rationale was that the individuals who had optimal comprehension (i.e., good-comprehenders) should have shown signs of more thorough syntactic processing during analysis of the sentences than poor-comprehenders. The findings confirmed that the good-comprehenders group had a greater syntactic-complexity-related negativity for the object-relative clauses than for the subject-relative clauses over the left frontal regions, whereas this was not the case in the poor-comprehenders group.

4.9 The Representation of Language(s) in the Multilingual Brain: Interpreters and Bilinguals

One of the more highly disputed matters in the cognitive neuroscience of language processing concerns the subject of multilingualism, in particular, how different languages are represented in the polyglot brain [55], and what degree of independence and/or interference exists across these languages. The search for a network of linguistic brain regions involved in the different aspects of language comprehension, reading, and production is complicated by several factors, such as the foreign language(s) and mother tongue proficiency levels, the age of acquisition of the foreign language(s) (since birth, within the 5th or 12th year, etc.), the modality and the time of exposure to the various linguistic contexts (e.g., at home, at school, at work), and the social-affective context of acquisition (e.g., within the family or at school), as well as the interactions among these factors [56].

Some studies support the notion that, given the same level of attained proficiency, there are not macroscopic differences in the way the different languages are processed by early fluent bilinguals, in particular there is no noticeable effect of the age of acquisition [57-59]. However, other studies provided evidence of remarkable differences in the time course of activation, and recruitment, of the neuroanatomical regions for linguistic analysis at different ages and in different cultural contexts [22, 56, 60-62]. The latter findings are consistent with the evidence that, although simultaneous interpreters proficiently master a foreign language, they always prefer to translate from that language into the mother tongue rather than from the latter into the former. They are also consistent with evidence indicating that simultaneous interpreters show a different pattern of hemispheric asymmetries during interpreting from and into the second language, in that there is a reduction of the left-sided lateralization of linguistic functions [63]. As previously stated, this difference between the mother tongue and the foreign language(s), linguistic proficiency being equal, is thought to be due to the fact that the mother tongue is learned contextually to the acquisition of conceptual knowledge (e.g., the notion about what a key /ki:/ is; that water /'wɔ:te(r)/ is a fresh liquid to drink) and to pragmatic world knowledge (e.g., that locked up doors cannot be opened; that the food is good /gʊd/, etc.). In other terms, the phonological form of the word is learned contextually to the acquisition of the conceptual contents. Conversely, the words of languages learned after the age of 5 years are somehow "translated" into the native language (i.e., "parasitism" according to Elizabeth Bates) to find a correspondence in the lexical system. This, clearly, would induce a significant difference in the ease of semantic access to the first language (L1) *vs* the second one (L2).

Electrophysiological evidence of this difference derives from an ERP study that we recently carried out on a group of professional simultaneous interpreters of the European Parliament [64]. These individuals represent a particular category of polyglots who have mastered several foreign languages clearly characterized by the age of acquisition. The interpreters in question mastered the English language, by means of which they interpreted for various organs of the European Community both from Italian into English and from English into Italian (both from Italian to English and vice versa, passive and active interpreting). They also had a less thorough knowledge of German (L3). The investigation of brain electrical activity in these interpreters allowed dissection of the effect of the age of acquisition of the mother tongue from that of the age of acquisition of the foreign language(s), independently of the proficiency factor. In this study, about 800 letter strings of a length varying between 6 and 10 characters, half of which were of low-frequency-use words (e.g., ECOGRAPHY or OBJECTION), were presented to a group of professional female interpreters of a mean age of 40 years. One-third of the strings were Italian words and non-words, while the other two-thirds consisted of English and German words and non-words.

4

The pseudo-words were clearly recognizable as belonging to a given language based on their orthographic appearance and legality. For instance, CHIUBANTO and DOIGNESCA were Italian pseudo-words, STIRBIGHT and SCROWFOND were English pseudo-words, and BERNSTACK and MEUSCHÄND were German pseudo-words. Similarly, the words were selected so that they would have an easily recognizable orthographic appearance. The task was of an orthographic nature and consisted in recognizing a given letter, announced by the experimenter at the beginning of each block of trials, which was or was not present in half of the trials in the administered string, and then responding accordingly by pushing a button. The interpreters did not need to care whether the string was a real word or a non-word in any of the languages. The findings showed a selection negativity to the target letter over the left occipital-temporal regions about 200 ms post-stimulus that was much greater for the mother tongue than for the foreign languages, hence revealing a strong effect of the age of acquisition. A negative component, consisting of a LPN (see Par. 4.6), was also observed over the frontal areas that was very sensitive to both language proficiency and age of acquisition. Such negativity, depicted in Fig. 4.10, was much

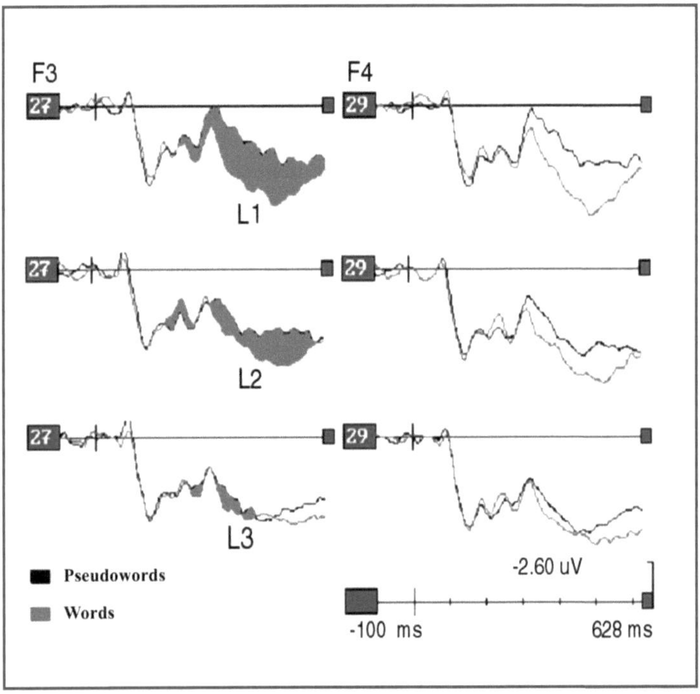

Fig. 4.10 Grand-average ERP waveforms recorded in professional simultaneous interpreters in response to words and pseudo-words of various languages (Italian= *L1*, English= *L2*, German= *L3*) at left (*F3*) and right (*F4*) frontal electrode sites. The *shaded area* represents the increased negativity in response to strings recognized as non-existent. Certainty about non-existence of a non-word diminishes as language proficiency decreases (L2 *vs* L3) and is much stronger for the mother tongue (L1) than for a foreign language (L2), independent of proficiency [64]

greater for pseudo-words than for words, indicating its sensitivity to word familiarity. What it is very interesting is that this negativity changed in amplitude as a function of the language for the pseudo-words too (i.e., items never seen before because they were non-existent), thus suggesting an influence of the differences in sensitivity to the orthographic appearance of L1 (Italian), L2 (English), and L3 (German). The LPN, and consequently the difference between the response to pseudo-words and words, was of larger amplitude for L1 than for L2, and for L2 than for L3. All in all, these effects proved to be robust signs of differences in proficiency across the foreign languages.

A thorough analysis of the interpreters' response to the German stimuli was also carried out, dividing them in two sub-groups: those who truly had a shallow knowledge of this language (non-fluent group) and those who considered it as a third language (L3) with respect to English but were nonetheless rather fluent in this language (fluent group). Examination of the changes in the LPN values as a function of the proficiency allowed a close investigation of the effects of mastering a foreign language. As seen in Fig. 4.11, the difference between pseudo-words and words was much greater for the fluent than for the non-fluent group, identifying the anterior LPN as a robustly predictive hallmark of the mastering of a foreign language.

Until this point, we have seen how ERPs might reveal the influence of the age of acquisition of a foreign language on brain responses to words and pseudo-words, even during a purely orthographic task. Thus, lexical access appears to be an automatic mechanism, and the advantage of the mother tongue, compared to the languages learned after the first five years of life, is essential.

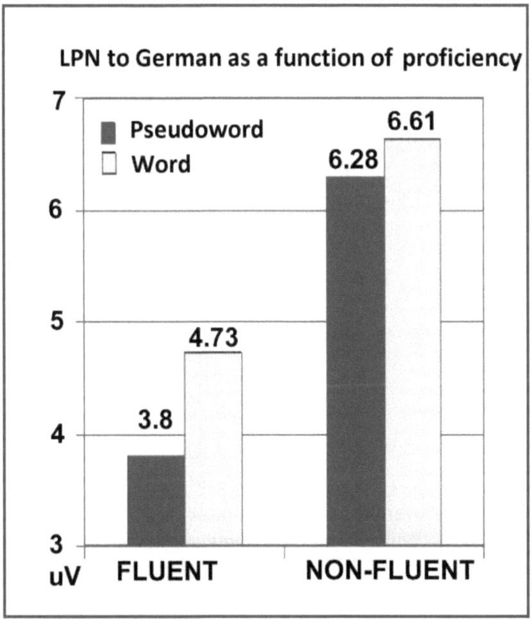

Fig. 4.11 Mean amplitude of the anterior LPN (in μV) recorded in response to words and non-words in professional interpreters as a function of their fluency in German (L3). Greater fluency is associated with a larger negativity for non-words, and therefore with a stronger lexical sensitivity

4

We now deal with another ERP component that has been shown to be sensitive to factors such as multilingualism in the syntactic analysis of linguistic stimuli, the syntactic P600. In a study carried out on early, fluent Italian/Slovenian bilinguals [22], we investigated the mechanisms of semantic and syntactic analyses by means of the terminal word paradigm. The task consisted in deciding whether the presented sentences were meaningful, or, for some reason, meaningless, with participants pushing one of two buttons with the index finger of the right or left hand, respectively. All the bilinguals who took part in the study lived in an area near Trieste, at the border between Italy and Slovenia, where a large Slovenian-speaking community resides within Italian territory. Hence, the language learned within the family and spoken at home and in the neighborhood was Slovenian (L1), whereas the language learned at school and spoken in the professional environment was mostly Italian (L2). We compared the group of bilinguals with a group of Italians, of similar mean age and cultural level, who lived in the same area but belonged to Italian families that were not acquainted with the Slovenian language. During the EEG recording, three types of sentences were presented to these individuals: correct sentences (e.g., "The light filtered through the SHUTTERS"), semantically incongruent sentences (e.g., "The structure of the city was too ENVIOUS"), or syntactically incongruent sentences (e.g., "He insisted because he wanted RELATING"). Along with 200 sentences in

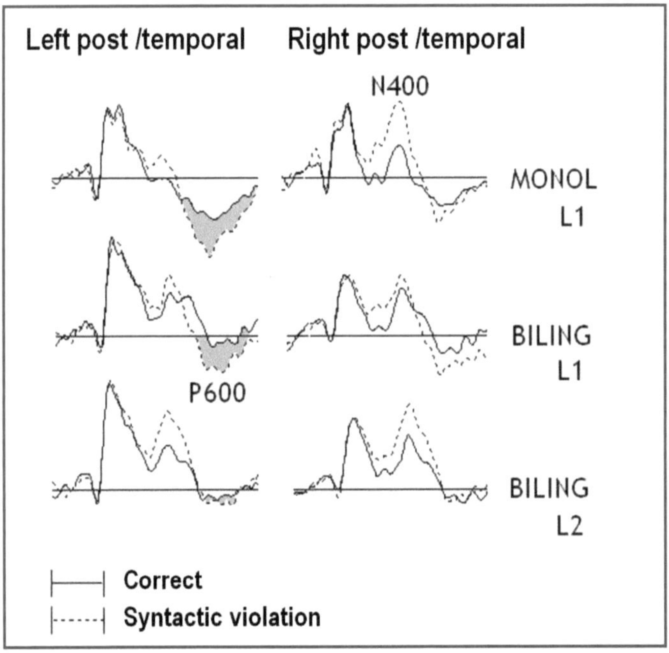

Fig. 4.12 Grand-average ERP waveforms recorded over the left and right posterior temporal regions in groups of Italian monolinguals and Italian/Slovenian fluent early bilinguals in response to correct or syntactically incongruent sentences. (Modified from Proverbio et al. [22], with the permission of MIT Press)

Italian, a similar number of sentences in Slovenian were presented, having a different meaning but balanced with respect to type. Among the most interesting of the highly variable findings was the detection of an orthographic N170 in the bilinguals that was mostly located over the left occipital-temporal cortex for L1, but which also extended toward the right homologous regions for L2, thus proving a lessening of the lateralization of the linguistic functions for L2 already at the orthographic analysis level. Similar findings were also obtained for the N400 and P600 components, reflecting overall a semantic and syntactic processing level, respectively.

As seen in Fig. 4.12, the N400 elicited by sentences that showed a syntactic violation, in addition to being semantically incongruent, exhibited the classic right-sided hemispheric topographic distribution in monolinguals. This asymmetry progressively decreased until becoming symmetrically bilateral in bilinguals for L2. As far as the latter syntactic analysis was concerned, at about 600 ms post-stimulus latency a positive component developed (Fig. 4.12). This positivity, which reflects secondary syntactic processes, was focused over the left temporal region in the monolinguals and was less lateralized for L1 (Slovenian) whereas it was clearly reduced in amplitude for L2 (Italian) in the bilinguals. All in all, these findings indicate the existence of macroscopic differences in the amplitude and topographic distribution of brain electrical activity as a function of both language proficiency and the social/affective context of its acquisition, whereas exposure to the language has a more marginal role.

In conclusion, it can be stated that ERPs are optimal temporal markers of mental processes subserving the mechanisms of language comprehension and reading.

References

1. Coltheart M, Rastle K, Perry C et al (2001) DRC: a dual route cascade model of visual word recognition and reading aloud. Psychol Review 108:204-256
2. Marshall JC, Newcombe F (1973) Patterns of paralexia: a psycholinguistic approach. J Psycholinguist Res 2:175-199
3. Temple CM, Marshall JC (1983) A case study of developmental phonological dyslexia. Br J Psychol 74: 517-533
4. Regan D (1989) Human brain electrophysiology: evoked potentials and evoked magnetic fields in science and medicine. Elsevier, New York
5. Zani A, Proverbio AM (eds) (2003) The cognitive electrophysiology of mind and brain. Academic Press/Elsevier, San Diego
6. Salmelin R (2007) Clinical neurophysiology of language: the MEG approach. Clin Neurophysiol 118:237-54
7. Kutas M (1987) Event-related brain potentials (ERPs) elicited during rapid serial visual presentation of congruous and incongruous sentences. EEG Clin Neurophysiol Suppl 40:406-411
8. Kutas M, Hillyard SA (1980) Reading senseless sentences: brain potentials reflect semantic incongruity. Science 11; 207:203-205
9. Cohen L, Dehaene S (2004) Specialization within the ventral stream: the case for the visual word form area. Neuroimage 22:466-476

4

10. Kronbichler M, Hutzler F, Wimmer H et al (2004) The visual word form area and the frequency with which words are encountered: evidence from a parametric fMRI study. Neuroimage 21:946-953
11. McCandliss BD, Cohen L, Dehaene S (2003) The visual word form area: expertise for reading in the fusiform gyrus. Trends Cogn Sci 7:293-299
12. Price CJ, Devlin JT (2004) The pro and cons of labelling a left occipitotemporal region: "the visual word form area". Neuroimage 22:477-479
13. Cohen L, Dehaene S, Naccache L et al (2000) The visual word form area. Spatial and temporal characterization of an initial stage of reading in normal subjects and posterior split-brain patients. Brain 123:291-307
14. Kuriki S, Takeuchi F, Hirata Y (1998) Neural processing of words in the human extrastriate visual cortex. Cogn Brain Res 6:193-203
15. Nobre AC, Allison T, McCarthy G (1994) Word recognition in the human inferior temporal lobe. Nature 372:260-263
16. Petersen SE, Fox PT, Posner M et al (1988) Positron emission tomographic studies of the cortical anatomy of single-word processing. Nature 331:585-589
17. Walla P, Endl W, Lindinger G et al (1999) Early occipito-parietal activity in a word recognition task: an EEG and MEG study. Clin Neurophysiol 10:1378-1387
18. Mechelli A, Gorno-Tempini ML, Price CJ (2003) Neuroimaging studies of word and pseudoword reading: consistencies, inconsistencies and limitations. J Cogn Neurosci 15:260-271
19. Bentin S, Mouchetant-Rostaing Y, Giard MH et al (1999) ERP manifestations of processing printed words at different psycholinguistic levels: time course and scalp distribution. J Cogn Neurosci 11:35-60
20. Helenius P, Tarkiainen A, Cornelissen P et al (1999) Dissociation of normal feature analysis and deficient processing of letter-strings in dyslexic adults. Cereb Cortex 9:476-483
21. Tarkiainen A, Helenius P, Hansen PC et al (1999) Dynamics of letter string perception in the human occipitotemporal cortex. Brain 122:2119-2132
22. Proverbio AM, Čok B, Zani A (2002) ERP measures of language processing in bilinguals. J Cogn Neurosci 14:994-1017
23. Proverbio AM, Vecchi L, Zani A (2004) From orthography to phonetics: ERP measures of grapheme-to-phoneme conversion mechanisms in reading. J Cogn Neurosci 16:301-317
24. Salmelin R, Helenius P, Service E (2000) Neurophysiology of fluent and impaired reading: a magnetoencephalographic approach. J Clin Neurophysiol 17:163-174
25. Shaywitz BA, Shaywitz SE, Pugh KR et al (2002) Disruption of posterior brain systems for reading in children with developmental dyslexia. Biol Psychiatry 52:101-110
26. Proverbio AM, Wiedemann F, Adorni R et al (2007) Dissociating object familiarity from linguistic properties in mirror word reading. Behav Brain Funct 3:43
27. Fiebach CJ, Friederici AD, Muller K, von Cramon DY (2002) fMRI evidence for dual routes to the mental lexicon in visual word recognition. J Cogn Neurosci 14:11-23
28. Rodriguez-Fornells A, Schmitt BM, Kutas M, Munte TF (2002) Electrophysiological estimates of the time course of semantic and phonological encoding during listening and naming. Neuropsychologia 40:778-787
29. Simos PG, Breier JI, Fletcher JM et al (2002) Brain mechanisms for reading words and pseudowords: an integrated approach. Cereb Cortex 12:297-305
30. Grossi G, Coch D, Coffey-Corina S et al (2001) Phonological processing in visual rhyming: a developmental ERP study. J Cogn Neurosci 13:610-625
31. Rugg MD, Barrett SE (1987) Event-related potentials and the interaction between orthographic and phonological information in a rhyme-judgment task. Brain Lang 32:336-361
32. Binder JR, Frost JA, Hammeke TA et al (2000) Human temporal lobe activation by speech and nonspeech sounds. Cereb Cortex 10:512-528

33. Proverbio AM, Zani A (2003) Time course of brain activation during graphemic/phonologic processing in reading: an ERP study. Brain Lang 87:412-420
34. Proverbio AM, Zani A (2005) Developmental changes in the linguistic brain after puberty. Trends Cogn Sci 9:164-167
35. Booth JR et al (2004) Development of brain mechanisms for processing orthographic and phonologic representations. J Cogn Neurosci 16:1234–1249
36. Mody M, Studdert-Kennedy M, Brady S (1997) Speech perception deficits in poor readers: auditory processing or phonological coding? J Exp Child Psychol 64:199-231
37. Serniclaes W, Sprenger-Charollcs L, Carre R, Demonet JF (2001) Perceptual discrimination of speech sounds in developmental dyslexia. J Speech Lang Hear Res 44:384-399
38. Näätänen R, Brattico E, Tervaniemi M (2003) Mismatch negativity (MMN): a probe to auditory cognition and perception in basic and clinical research. In: Zani A, Proverbio AM (eds) The cognitive electrophysiology of mind and brain. Academic Press, San Diego
39. Kujala T, Naatanen R (2001) The mismatch negativity in evaluating central auditory dysfunction in dyslexia. Neurosci Biobehav Rev 25:535-543
40. Leppanen PH, Pihko E, Eklund KM, Lyytinen H (1999) Cortical responses of infants with and without a genetic risk for dyslexia: II. Group effects. Neuroreport 10:969-973
41. King JW, Kutas M (1998) Neural plasticity in the dynamics of human visual word recognition. Neurosci Lett 244:616-614
42. Schendan HE, Ganis G, Kutas M (1998) Neurophysiological evidence for visual perceptual categorization of words and faces within 150 ms. Psychophysiology 35:240-251
43. Assadollahi R, Pulvermüller F (2003) Early influences of word length and frequency: a group study using MEG. Neuroreport 14:1183-1187
44. Pulvermüller F, Assadollahi R, Elbert T (2001) Neuromagnetic evidence for early semantic access in word recognition. Eur J Neurosci 13:201-205
45. Johnson R Jr (1986) A triarchic model of P300 amplitude. Psychophysiology 23:367-384
46. Donchin E (1987) The P300 as a metric for mental workload. EEG Clin Neurophysiol Suppl 39:338-343
47. Van Berkum JJA, Hagoort P, Brown CM (1999) Semantic integration in sentences and discourse: evidence from the N400. J Cogn Neurosci 11:657-671
48. Hagoort P, Hald L, Bastiaansen M, Petersson KM (2004) Integration of word meaning and world knowledge in language comprehension. Science 304:438-441
49. Friederici AD (2002) Towards a neural basis of auditory sentence processing. Trends Cogn Sci 6:78–84
50. Friederici AD (1995)The time course of syntactic activation during language processing: a model based on neuropsychological and neurophysiological data. Brain Lang 50:259–281
51. Münte TF, Heinze HJ, Mangun GR (1993) Dissociation of brain activity related to syntactic and semantic aspects of language. J Cogn Neurosci 5:335–344
52. Osterhout L, Holcomb PJ (1992) Event-related brain potentials elicited by syntactic anomaly. J Memory Lang 31:785–806
53. Hagoort P (2003) How the brain solves the binding problem for language: a neurocomputational model of syntactic processing. NeuroImage 20:18-29
54. Federmeier KD, Kluender R, Kutas M (2002) Aligning linguistic and brain views on language comprehension, In: Zani A, Proverbio AM (eds) The cognitive electrophysiology of mind and brain. Academic Press, San Diego
55. Hernandez A, Li P, MacWhinney B (2005) The emergence of competing modules in bilingualism. Trends Cogn Sci 9:220-225
56. Proverbio AM, Adorni R, Zani A (2007) The organization of multiple languages in polyglots: interference or independence? J Neuroling 20:25-49
57. Illes J, Francis WS, Desmond JE et al (1999) Convergent cortical representation of semantic processing in bilinguals. Brain Lang 70:347-363

4

58. Paradis M (1996) Selective deficit in one language is not a demonstration of different anatomical representation. Comments on Gomez-Tortosa et al (1995). Brain Lang 54:170-173
59. Perani D, Abutalebi J (2005) The neural basis of first and second language processing. Current Opin Neurobiol 15:202-206
60. Roux FE, Lubrano V, Lauwers-Cances V et al (2004) Intra-operative mapping of cortical areas involved in reading in mono- and bilingual patients. Brain 127:1796-1810
61. Dehaene S, Dupoux E, Mehler J et al (1997) Anatomical variability in the cortical representation of first and second language. Neuroreport 8:3809-3815
62. Lucas TH, McKhann GM, Ojemann GA (2004) Functional separation of languages in the bilingual brain: a comparison of electrical stimulation language mapping in 25 bilingual patients and 117 monolingual control patients. J Neurosurg 101:449-457
63. Fabbro F, Gran L, Basso G, Bava A (1990) Cerebral lateralization in simultaneous interpretation. Brain Lang 39:69-89
64. Proverbio AM, Adorni R, Del Zotto M, Zani A (2005) The effect of age of acquisition and proficiency on language-related brain activation in interpreters: an ERP study. Psychophysiology 42(S1):S7

Section II
Neuropragmatics. Psychophysiological, Neuropsychological and Cognitive Correlates

From Pragmatics to Neuropragmatics 5

M. Balconi, S. Amenta

5.1 Communication and Pragmatics

Two metaphors coined by Reddy [1], the *conduit metaphor* and the *toolmaker's paradigm*, can be used to introduce several observations on the nature of communication and its pragmatic properties. The conduit metaphor depicts linguistic expression as channels carrying ideas and meanings: mental representations are poured into the conduit and are extracted from it, without undergoing modifications. Seen in this light, communication is nothing more than the exchange of information among individuals. The toolmaker's paradigm, by contrast, explains communication through a more complex scenario, in which speakers live in distant worlds; no one knows anything about their language, culture, and characteristics, and the only means of communication is through the exchange of blueprints of tools. Inhabitants of these worlds are proud of their projects and are disappointed when they are misunderstood. In fact, it is reason enough to rejoice when, on occasion, the blueprints are received correctly, without further specifications.

These metaphors represent two ideas of communication, but while the first appears to be a superficial description of communicative processes, the second actually reflects how human communication works. Communicative messages can be thought of as blueprints, projects which can be interpreted in multiple ways and that bring no guarantee of their correct interpretation. Many factors and variables are involved in interpreting messages and only a few are directly controlled by the speaker alone. Furthermore, this perspective suggests that messages are the product of a "building" process, which implies strategic choices and assumptions regarding the interlocutor's beliefs and representations.

M. Balconi (✉)
Department of Psychology, Catholic University of Milan, Milan, Italy

5

Accordingly, two topics become fundamental: first of all we must define the notion of pragmatic meaning and its relation to the concepts, mental representations, and cognitive processes (representations, planning, intentions) from which it originates. Second, we need to explore the relationship between semantics (the study of meaning) and pragmatics (the study of language use) [2, 3].

5.1.1 "Pragmatic Meaning" and the Semantics/Pragmatics Interface

The main question is: what is meaning [4-6]? Although meaning is often represented as a property of words or sentences, and therefore is studied only as such, pragmatics acknowledges a wider domain for meaning, one which permeates human life and activities. Meaning is linked to actions and to intentions: successful communication has to be seen as a process that aims to realize a condition of mutual knowledge relative to a communicative intention. From a pragmatics perspective, meaning is more than the composition of single linguistic units and their meanings, as it must be defined by considering what speakers intend to communicate and what listeners are able to comprehend through inferential processes [7]. Therefore, pragmatic meaning is constructed in the interaction between rational individuals endowed with intentionality and beliefs about the world and bearers of a *Weltanaschauung* that can frame and shape the interpretation and production of messages. Thus, the analysis of meaning cannot disregard intentionality, choices, representations, and inferences.

The second question we need to address is: what is the relationship between semantics and pragmatics? There is general agreement on a substantial separation of the two disciplines (and the functions they study): pragmatics studies the meaning of utterances, that is, *what is meant* by the speaker or how the speaker uses language in order to pursuit his or her communicative intention; semantics studies the meanings of word and sentences, assuming meaning to be a composite property of the meanings of the individual words and sentences. Thus, both disciplines study the meaning of linguistic expression, but while semantics focuses on linguistic expression itself, pragmatics deals with the processes activated by speakers in the construction of mutual states of knowledge.

Nonetheless, pragmatics cannot be limited to the study of how speakers add contextual information to linguistic structures in order to convey/withdraw meanings. Pragmatic function goes far beyond the simple summing up of information, and pragmatics should be defined as the study of the processes actuated by an individual endowed with a complex *cognitive* and *emotional choice* that can be applied to fulfill the mutual exchange of meanings.

5.2 Pragmatic Issues

5.2.1 The Origins of Pragmatic Perspective

What is pragmatics really? It is not simple to find a unique definition, basically due to the plurality of processes involved in what is commonly called "pragmatic competence" and to the interdisciplinarity of pragmatics as a branch of the linguistic and communicative sciences. Traditionally, the object of investigation in pragmatics has been confined to *language use*, specifically, the study of the use of language and the study of language as a means for human action. In other words, pragmatics can be defined as an examination of how individuals involved in social/communicative interactions produce/convey and receive/understand the meaning of what is said through language; in other words, language from the point of view of its properties and processes of use [8].

But how did we arrive at this representation? The current definition of pragmatics derives from Morris's theories [9] on communication. Morris considered pragmatics as the "relation between signs and interpreters." According to this theory, pragmatics follows both semantics, as the study of the relation between signs and objects (referents), and syntax, as the study of the relation between signs. However, further theories have been formulated based on the relation between signs and users. In particular, Grice [10] focused on how speakers are able to pursue a specific communicative intent and how listeners can recognize it by elaborating a complex system of rules based on the *principle of cooperation*. Austin and Searle [11, 12], on the other hand, adopting the principle that "speaking is acting," sought to classify communicative intentions, thus elaborating the concept of *speech acts*.

5.2.2 Pragmatic Competence as Communicative "Strategy" and "Option"

Complementary theory, which considers pragmatics as an additional linguistic component (along with phonologic, morphosyntactic, and semantic components [9]), has gradually been overshadowed by new theories addressing pragmatic competence as a fundamental aspect of a more general communicative competence [13]. Following this approach, any level of communicative and linguistic production can be studied from a pragmatic perspective, such that the question becomes: what do people do when using language? Or, what do they do through language? In fact, when producing and comprehending communicative messages, individuals are actively engaged in different cognitive tasks, all aimed at fulfilling a complex communicative goal. Therefore, the study of language usage cannot be limited to the cognitive processes involved in integrating different kinds of information (as is done in classical definitions of pragmatics) but instead requires a study of the means by which individuals modulate and regulate all possible linguistic levels in order to achieve their communicative intentions.

In particular, using language to communicate engages individuals in continuous processes of decision-making about linguistic options. As noted above, these choices concern any of the linguistic components: phonetics, phonologic, morphologic, syntactic, lexical, and semantic. In the first place, these choices are made at a structural level (e.g., giving a particular syntactic form to a sentence); in the second place, pragmatic choices involve communicative strategies. This perspective allows us to re-formulate the classical definition of pragmatics, focusing now on the cognitive processes that make communication possible more than on the communicative rules [13, 14]. Intrinsic to this decision-making process are several principles that concur to define the nature of pragmatic competence. In particular, individuals make choices and build strategies based on some of the unique properties of pragmatic/communicative competence, such as:

- *variability*: the property of communication that defines the range of communicative possibilities, among which is formulating communicative choices;
- *negotiability*: the possibility of making choices based on flexible strategies;
- *adaptability*: the ability to modulate and regulate communicative choices in relation to the communicative context;
- *salience*: the degree of awareness reached by communicative choices;
- *indeterminacy*: the possibility to re-negotiate pragmatic choices as the interaction unfolds in order to fulfill communicative intentions;
- *dynamicity*: development of the communicative interaction in time.

5.2.3 Pragmatics, Comprehension and Inference

Regarding comprehension, pragmatics addresses especially the chain of inferences that allows individuals to understand communicative messages [14]. Comprehending meaning, from a pragmatic perspective, requires listeners to perform two basic tasks: decoding what is said (semantic meaning) and understanding what is meant (pragmatic meaning) [10, 15, 16]. That is, pragmatic theories agree in considering meaning as comprising a semantic component (the meaning of what is said) and a pragmatic component (the meaning derived by what is intended by the speaker). Both the process involved in the unification of the two components and the time-course of these processes are, however, still subjects of debate.

Classical pragmatic theories have identified three levels of meaning: literal/minimum meaning, what is said, what is meant. Different explanations have been given about how individuals are able to integrate the three levels [10, 16-18]. Among these, Grice [10] suggested that human communication is founded on the *cooperative principle* (CP), constraining speakers and listeners to follow certain communicative maxims (quality, quantity, relation, manner) which, in turn, allow for the correct conveyance and decoding of communicative intents. Starting from this assumption, *what is said* overlaps with the minimum literal meaning of a sentence, while in order to understand *what is meant* it is necessary to draw inferences about the speaker's mental state (*conversational implicatures*). Expanding Grice's considerations, some authors [16, 17] have extended pragmatic processes to the determination of what is said; thus, meanings not derived from linguistic decoding (e.g., reference assignment) are built by adding pragmatic knowledge to the unfolding proposition.

Finally, a further extension of the role of pragmatic processes has been made by relevance theorists [15, 19]: pragmatic processes concern the determination of both what is said and what is meant. According to *relevance theory*, the main aim of inferential pragmatics is to detect communicative intentions and the meaning of what speakers *intend* to communicate. In other words, the linguistic code is not sufficient to determine the totality of what is explicitly expressed by a sentence (*under-determinacy thesis*); therefore, in order to reconstruct what is communicated by the speaker, the listener must carry out cognitive inferential processes guided by pragmatic principles. Moreover, linguistic encoding processes do not aim to maximize explicitness, but to reduce the cognitive effort required by the decoding process. Communication is therefore guided by *cognitive* and *communicative principles of relevance* (see [15]), which are to be considered as the direct function of the cognitive effects conveyed through the message and the indirect function of the cognitive effort required to infer the intended meaning.

5.2.4
Pragmatics and Context: Salience and the Direct Access View

As noted above, the role of contextual elements in determining a speaker's meaning is a crucial point in pragmatics. Experimental pragmatics, adopting psycholinguistic methodologies–implemented, most of the time, using neuropsychological measures (such as EEG and ERPs, see Chapter 2)–specifically addresses integration of the linguistic and contextual elements of a message [19]. Two different hypotheses can be considered as representative of the two approaches that elucidate the relation language/context: the *graded salience hypothesis* [20] and the *direct access view* [21, 22].

The first hypothesis, formulated by Giora, considers pragmatic information as secondary to semantic information, which is processed earlier. Giora suggested the existence of two different mechanisms for processing linguistic messages: one is dedicated to linguistic information and the other to contextual information. The first mechanism is responsible for lexical access and is activated by the information encoded within the mental lexicon on the basis of salience. The second is sensitive to contextual information and operates to construct the global meaning of a message. The two mechanisms are separate but operate in parallel. Priority access is given to salient meanings. To be salient, a meaning should be encoded in the mental lexicon; this happens on the basis of its frequency, prototypicality, conventionality, and familiarity. It is only when salient meanings are contextually incompatible that further inferential processes, involving the elaboration of contextual information, are activated.

The second hypothesis, according to the model proposed by Gibbs, predicts an earlier interaction of linguistic and contextual information in order to obtain a complete representation of what is meant by the speaker. Thus, according to the direct access view, there is only one mechanism responsible for the elaboration of linguistic and non-linguistic information; moreover, linguistic and contextual information interact early on to ensure the construction of contextually appropriate meanings and the inhibition of contextually inappropriate meanings. In other words, when given enough contextual information, listeners are able to directly access the correct interpretation of what is said, without elaborating conventional (but not appropriate) sentence meanings.

5.3 Neuropragmatics

5.3.1 The Neuropragmatic Perspective

If pragmatics deals mostly with the uses of language, neuropragmatics aims to analyze the relation between brain structures and functions on the one hand, and the mental processes involved in language use on the other. The neuropragmatic perspective is concerned with the modalities used by healthy or damaged brains to produce and understand communicative messages [23, 24]. In particular, neuropragmatics, by investigating cerebral activity through a multicomponential approach, integrates the methodologies and models of linguistic and cognitive pragmatics with neurolinguistics, cognitive neuroscience, and experimental neuropsychology. Its principal goals are: (1) to establish itself as a paradigm with which to test pragmatic theories through the use of advanced technologies (e.g., brain imaging) and (2) to investigate the neural basis of the cognitive processes involved in communication, intended as an intentional and finalized action and as a complex cognitive process oriented to the construction and sharing of meanings.

Using data collected from healthy and clinical populations, neuropragmatics acknowledges two principal branches: *clinical neuropragmatics*, dealing with deficits in production/comprehension of specific components of communicative processes [25-27], and *cognitive neuropragmatics*, which investigates pragmatic abilities as sequences of mental states entertained in order to design and understand communicative acts. The neuropragmatic study of language consists of an analysis of the neural basis of pragmatic abilities; that is, which networks are activated and in which timeframes. The focus of neuropragmatics is on the complexity of communication, which, as a cognitive process, involves a plurality of cognitive functions (memory, attention, monitoring, consciousness, perception, etc.). These are in turn integrated and synchronized to achieve the production and comprehension of linguistic and extralinguistic acts and to allow their regulation as a function of the speaker's plans and scope.

5.3.2
Neuropragmatic Issues

In the majority of neuropragmatic studies, either the deficits of pragmatic abilities in a brain-damaged population are described [28-32], or pragmatic meanings have been elaborated in healthy samples [33-36]. Here, we have thus far explored concerns regarding the representation of pragmatic function, and specifically its explication within distinct *brain networks* or *modules*. There is still no general agreement on whether there is a specific module dedicated to the representation of cognitive processes involved in linguistic and communicative acts. In fact, the modular hypothesis has been gradually substituted by hypotheses in which distributed networks interface with and integrate a plurality of systems and functions involved in pragmatic production and the comprehension of language [37, 38].

However, a second issue concerns the problem of *integrating theories* and *methodologies* coming from the different fields of analysis [39]. For neuropragmatic studies in particular, it is possible to recognize a substantial asymmetry in production/comprehension analyses. In fact, studies on language comprehension have focused on figurative language, indirect communication, and inferential processes; while production studies have concentrated on discourse abilities and deficits in clinical populations. In this regard, an integrated view of pragmatic processes is still in progress.

Definitely linked with these two open issues and partially a derivation of classical neuropsychology is a third issue, which concerns the "time" and "place" of pragmatic processes. Acceptance of right brain dominance for pragmatic processes [40, 41] is progressively being replaced by interest in the role of the frontal lobes in the elaboration of pragmatic abilities [42]. Serious attention is also being paid to the development of pragmatic processes in the timeline of language comprehension.

The next paragraph of this chapter aim to explore the neuropragmatic approach to communication by considering irony as a case study.

5.4
Irony Elaboration: Definition, Models and Empirical Evidence

Figurative language is one of the main focuses of neuropragmatics. Metaphors, idioms (see Chapter 4), general non-compositional strings (see Chapter 5), and irony have been studied using different methodologies, such as functional magnetic resonance imaging (fMRI) and event-related potentials (ERPs) along with classical lesion studies in clinical populations. The reasons for the emphasis placed by neuropragmatic on figurative language lie in the processes necessary to grasp non-explicit meanings. If inferential processes are operative in simple linguistic functions (e.g., reference assignation) and more complex discourse processes (i.e., co-reference, coherence), in figurative language they become particularly apparent. When a person says: "This bag weighs tons" it is immediately clear to the listener that the speaker is using hyperbole, since a bag cannot weigh tons, it is just very heavy and difficult to carry. Things become more complex when individuals are faced with more articulated or ambiguous sentences, as may happen with irony. Think of the following situation: two friends are rushing to get to work in time for a very important meeting. Both of them are well-dressed and carrying a cup of coffee. One of them, while walking, inadvertently hits the other, causing the latter to slosh hot brown liquid on his white shirt. The second man says: (a) "Oh, pay attention next time. What a disaster!" (b) "Oh, thank you!" or (c) "That's just perfect!" While in (a) the speaker is being quite explicit, in (b) and (c) he is clearly expressing something other than what he is actually uttering. Irony is quite apparent in (b) and (c); however, whereas many of the sentences people utter commonly are ironic, irony is difficult to define.

From its classical Greek etymology *eironeia*, modern definitions of irony have referred to aspects relating to dissimulation and derision; thus, speakers are using irony when they hide what they are thinking and pretend to think something else in order to mock someone or something. But there is more to irony than simple *pretence*. Generally, it is possible to define irony as a pragmatic phenomenon whose intended meaning (*figurative*) is opposite to the expressed meaning (*literal*). However, different theories have tried to define irony by focusing on its different features. Thus, it has been described as a form of *semantic anomaly* [10, 11] and as a *pragmatic anomaly* [43, 44]. Cognitive approaches have considered irony as a particular *figure of thought* [45-47] appealing to the concept of *counterfactuality*. Finally, communicative approaches have addressed irony as a *discommunication phenomenon* involving the representation of different levels of complex communicative intentions.

The complexity of understanding irony seems to be due to the presence of the multiple intentions guiding ironic communication. In fact, when an utterance is consistent with the state of the world it represents or with contextual expectations, as in (a), it is easy to comprehend the speaker's intentions. But when a sentence is not congruent with the context it is uttered in, then different possibilities open up: the speaker is lying, or she/he is mistaken, or she/he is being ironic. Furthermore, most of the time irony is not expressed by clear contrasts as in (b) and (c), since ironic meaning may be committed to different forms of speech, such as hyperbole or understatement (e.g., "Looks like I stained my shirt") [48]. Sometimes, irony is conveyed through sentences that are true but which are not consistent with the situation they refer to ("I see you are always very careful around hot cups") [47, 49].

To recognize and understand communicative intentions beyond such complex utterances, certain meta-representational abilities are necessary. In fact, when faced with ironic sentences, listeners have to integrate semantic knowledge relative to what has been said with contextual knowledge (situational elements, world knowledge, hypotheses on the speaker's state of mind and his or her emotional states). The two kinds of information are referred to, in pragmatics, as *local* and *global* factors. One of the main issues in irony comprehension concerns when and how the cognitive system integrates local and global information in order to re-construct ironic meaning.

Models on irony comprehension will be discussed in the next paragraph, while Par. 5.4.2 deals with empirical evidence.

5.4.1 Models of Irony Understanding

Pragmatic discussions of figurative language comprehension in general, and irony in particular, have still not reached a definitive answer to the question how an individual understands utterances that go beyond their literal meaning? Thus far, three hypotheses have been broadly accredited: the *standard pragmatic hypothesis* [10, 11], the *parallel access model* [50, 51], and the above-mentioned *direct access view* [18, 52].

Standard pragmatics assumes that irony is to be considered, along with other forms of figurative language, as a violation of conversational maxims, in particular as a violation of the quantity maxim. Thus, ironic meaning results from a falsification of the sentence's literal meaning via contextual information. In order to understand irony, it is therefore necessary to acknowledge the speaker's real intentions and meanings beyond what is said. To do so, it is *first* necessary to recognize that the speaker means something else, and *then* re-construct the figurative meaning, which is usually the opposite of what is said. Standard pragmatics hypothesizes that a listener first computes the literal meaning, then tests this meaning against reality, and, in case it is found context-incongruent, computes a new meaning that is compatible with the situation. The process operating to re-construct a speaker's meanings requires complex inferential processes (the conversational implicatures referred to in Par. 5.2.3), thus recruiting more cognitive resources, as indexed by longer elaboration times [50, 53]. However, standard pragmatic assumptions have been challenged by data showing that ironic and non-ironic elaboration are of the same length [18], as proposed by parallel access models (in some cases) and the direct access view. According to parallel access models, access is gained by both the literal and the ironic meaning of an ironic sentence and the two are elaborated in parallel. The two principal models referring to this approach are the *graded salience hypothesis* (see Par. 5.2.4) [20] and the *parallel race mode* [51, 54].

Giora [20] suggested that salient meanings are processed with priority. Familiar and conventional ironies have two salient meanings: literal and ironic. In this case, therefore, the order in which the meanings are processed is a function of their grade of salience. If the figurative meaning is less salient than the literal meaning, it will be granted secondary access, whereas if the literal meaning is less salient than the ironic meaning, then the latter will be processed earlier.

In parallel, Dews and Winner [51], developing the hypothesis formulated by Long and Graesser [54], proposed that the literal and ironic meanings of ironic sentences are always activated and remain operative so that listeners can perceive the irony of a message and thus derive the intended meaning. Both meanings are therefore contemporaneously accessed and concurrently processed. This model found confirmation in a recent clinical study [55], in which pragmatically impaired patients were asked to process ironic endings of stories. Those patients, though unable to recognize the irony of the endings, were able to understand their literal meaning, thus providing evidence that the literal meanings were active.

A third approach assumes, in particular cases, that ironic meanings obtain direct access [18, 56]. Gibbs suggested that a context providing enough information allows

5

Table 5.1 Principal psycholinguistic models of irony comprehension and ERP predictions

Pragmatic model	Irony elaboration hypothesis	Related ERP effects
Standard Pragmatics (Grice, 1975)	- Priority of lexical semantic information - Ironic meaning is derived after literal meaning has been rejected as the intended meaning	- N400 effect (semantic anomaly detection)
Graded Salience (Giora, 2003)	- Priority of salient meanings over contextual fit - Activation and processing of both meanings for familiar ironies; processing of the only salient meaning (literal) for non familiar ironies	- N400 effect for non familiar ironies - Late ERPs effect for familiar ironies (meaning selection)
Direct Access (Gibbs, 1994; 2002)	- Priority of contextual information - Early interaction of lexical-semantic and contextual information to select context compatible meanings - Direct access of ironic meanings	- No N400 effect - No late ERPs effect

for the direct and automatic figurative interpretation of sentences, i.e., without the need for a first phase of literal processing. In fact, when sufficient contextual information is present, the figurative meaning of ironic sentences becomes conventional, while elaboration of the literal meaning becomes optional and unnecessary. This hypothesis has been tested through a reading time paradigm, whose basic assumptions suggest that sentence reading times reflect elaboration processes. Longer reading times indicate that a sentence requires more complex and effortful elaboration processes, while shorter reading times indicate a lessened cognitive effort for the elaboration. Reading times of non-conventional ironic sentences reflected the greater cognitive effort required to process ironic meanings compared to literal ones, while reading times were the same for literal sentences and conventional ironies [50, 53, 57]. Table 5.1 provides a synthesis of the proposed models.

5.4.2 Irony Comprehension: Empirical Contributions

5.4.2.1 ERP Studies

The ability of ERPs to measure electrical brain activity with a high temporal resolution explains their immense usefulness in neuropragmatic studies aimed at investigating the time course of language (literal and figurative) processing (see Chapter 2). A number of ERP studies have focused on figurative language comprehension, such as metaphors [58-61] and idioms (see Chapter 7). Most of these studies have evidenced a greater amplitude of the N400 component in response to figurative sentences than to literal sentences, suggesting that semantic elaboration is more difficult during figurative language comprehension.

The results of ERP studies on irony are conflicting, probably attributable to the plurality of methodologies involved and to differences in the paradigms used. A recent study [62] reported that the N400 amplitude was higher when subjects were asked to focus on sentence plausibility (holistic strategy) during the processing of ironic sentences than under analytical conditions, in which subjects were required to focus on the congruence of words within the sentence. The N400 effect has been related to difficulties in establishing the semantic meaning of ironies, due to the fact that no sufficient contextual information has been provided. Cornejo and colleagues reported the presence of a late positivity in the pattern of ironic interpretation compared to literal sentences, associated with a larger demand of cognitive resources for closure processes aimed at establishing global semantic coherence and plausibility. The N400 effect was not reported, however, in another study comparing literal, ironic, and counterfactual ironic sentences through an auditory modality [63], suggesting that the processing of ironic sentences is not different from the processing of literal sentences, at least at a semantic level. Those results were confirmed by a recent study [64] in which endings to literal and ironic stories were compared. The authors reported that, along with the absence of an N400 component, there was a posterior P600 effect, which has been related to pragmatic processes of global coherence attribution.

These data seem to indicate that ironic and literal comprehension processes are similar in early phases, while some differences are detected in later time windows. With respect to the traditional model presented in the previous paragraph, we can say the standard pragmatics hypothesis has been ruled out since no N400 effect, indicating a semantic anomaly recognition process, has been found. Nonetheless, the data also seem unable to endorse the direct access view, since late effects have been recorded. In conclusion, ERP data suggest that irony elaboration does not pose a problem in terms of semantic elaboration. However, the definition of ironic meanings may require the need to invoke further processes, in an aim to re-establish the global coherence and plausibility of sentence representation.

5.4.2.2
Clinical Neuropsychology Studies

Clinical studies seek to identify the cognitive processes and brain areas involved in irony elaboration. Most studies have focused on the relation between comprehension and brain lesions, in an effort to individuate the neural networks necessary for pragmatic comprehension. Studies on irony and sarcasm comprehension emphasize the role of the right hemisphere [65-67] and frontal areas [68-70] in ironic decoding.

The right hemisphere is active in the mediation of visual-spatial and non-verbal functions (see Chapter 1). In particular, it is primarily involved, within the paralinguistic domain, in modulation of the acoustic and prosodic components of communication [71]. Moreover, patients with damage to the right hemisphere (RBD) show general pragmatic impairments associated with, for instance, figurative language comprehension (metaphors, idioms, proverbs, and humor) [32, 72-74] and prosodic modulation control, thus resulting in deficits in the usage of prosodic indexes in language production and comprehension [75-77].

Tompkins and Mateers [78] investigated the ability of RBDs regarding sarcastic sentence comprehension. Subjects were required to listen to paired acoustic stimuli (script descriptions), one modulated with a positive prosody and the other uttered with a negative prosody. Stimuli always represented positive scenarios, therefore making the positive inflection congruent and the negative inflection non-congruent with context expectations. The authors reported that the subjects had difficulties in integrating ironic/non-congruent endings with the previous story context, due mostly to difficulties in identifying the correct prosody of the test sentences. It was concluded that the deficits of RBDs in irony comprehension may be due to impairments in prosodic elaboration and usage.

More recently, Winner and colleagues [68] conducted an experiment investigating the ability of RBDs to correctly infer mental states. The authors used scripts comparable to those used in the Tompkins and Mateers experiment [78], but instead of modulating prosodic elements they manipulated the character of the information describing the situation represented in the script such that the final comment of these scripts could have been interpreted as ironic—assuming subjects were able to identify a state of mutual knowledge relative to the story's character—or as a lie. The authors reported a higher number of mistakes in irony detection, attributable to difficulties in assessing the speaker's mutual knowledge.

Globally, clinical studies have highlighted the role of the right hemisphere concerning the non-verbal components of irony, which have the basic function of marking ironic communication and expressing affective attitudes. In addition, lesions studies have evidenced the role of meta-representational processes involving especially the frontal lobes.

5.4.2.3
Neuroimaging Studies

Neuroimaging techniques such as fMRI are hemodynamic measures of brain activity and have a high spatial resolution. They can therefore provide information about the brain areas and circuits involved in processing the pragmatic aspects of language.

Ironic discourse endings were recently investigated in an experiment that compared literal, metaphoric, and ironic language comprehension [79]. Ironic sentences produced an increased activity of the right superior and middle temporal gyri, attributed to processes aimed at establishing the coherence of ironic sentences with regard to contextual information. Moreover, the data showed distinct pathways of activation for irony, metaphors, and literal remarks, thus confirming hypotheses about the existence of different neurocognitive processes involved in comprehending different forms of figurative language. In the right hemisphere, higher activation for irony has been associated with processes relevant to coherent discourse representation. By contrast, increased activation in the left inferior gyrus and inferior temporal regions for metaphors has been related to more effortful semantic selection [79].

Furthermore, the successful understanding of irony has been found to involve mentalizing abilities, as we observed from clinical neuropsychological studies. Uchiyama and colleagues [80] reported that the comprehension of ironic remarks elicited larger activation of the medial prefrontal cortex, associated with theory of mind processes. Their results indicated that some kind of mentalizing process is necessary in order to comprehend ironic meaning. Moreover, increased activation of the left inferior prefrontal gyrus, as reported by the same authors, has been associated with extra activity due to the interaction of linguistic and mentalizing processes during irony detection.

Recently, a developmental study investigated the acquisition of pragmatic abilities relative to ironic sentences and sought to identify the neural basis of irony elaboration processes [81]. The experiment compared children and adult performances in irony detection and comprehension by using cartoon-stories that presented simple conventional interactions, involving ironic or non-ironic remarks (presented acoustically with an ironic or non-ironic prosody). In the experiment, the affective elements related to prosody and to facial expression were explicit. The authors reported increased activation of the medial prefrontal cortex in both adults and children in response to ironic sentences. This result has been attributed to integration of the affective information conveyed by facial expression and prosody. Moreover, right hemisphere was strongly activated under ironic conditions, thus confirming the hypothesis of a dominant role for the right hemisphere in ironic decoding [32, 78], particularly regarding the integration of contextual indexes aimed at comprehension of the discourse level [82]. However, the data also showed different pathways of activation for adults and children. Adults presented higher activity of the right fusiform cortex, a region associated with the elaboration of facial and emotional expressions [83], and of the striate cortex. This result suggests that adult tend to focus their attention on facial expressions and to use them heuristically to infer intended meanings. In children, by contrast, there was increased activation of the prefrontal regions associated with mentalizing processes. It is therefore possible that interactive and communicative experience enforces the individual's ability to decode complex meaning, so that while children still need to engage in complex inferential procedures based on mentalizing activity, adults can rely on non-verbal indexes, and infer directly the type of interaction in which they are involved.

The combined use of increasingly sophisticated technologies has allowed exploration of the multiplicity of processes involved in irony with higher resolution and precision, thus providing a more complete picture of what happens when individuals are faced with complex communicative contexts.

Through the neuropragmatic approach, studies have been able to individuate the cognitive processes and their neural basis during ironic decoding, to establish the time course of ironic meaning construction, and to observe the effects of different

5

cognitive strategies in the process of comprehension. Moreover, they have granted insight into the development of comprehension in interactive contexts, by taking into account linguistic and emotional components simultaneously.

These results seem to indicate that the comprehension of irony does not require special semantic processes (absence of the N400 ERP effect), while late processes of pragmatic revision aiming to construct discourse coherence seem to be essential to the derivation of ironic meanings. ERPs results have been confirmed by neuroimaging studies showing greater activation of the brain areas involved in mentalizing and in decision-making processes (prefrontal cortex). Moreover, neuroimaging studies have indicated that the integration of verbal and non-verbal components, linked to emotional aspects of irony, are crucial for irony comprehension, especially in adults, as was previously suggested in lesion studies.

References

1. Reddy MJ (1979) The conduit metaphor - a case of frame conflict in our language about language. In: Ortony A (ed) Metaphor and thought. Cambridge University Press, London, pp 284-324
2. Szabo ZC (ed) (2005) Semantics versus pragmatics. Oxford University Press, New York
3. Jaszczolt KM (2002) Semantics and pragmatics. Longman, London
4. Peirce CS (1894) What is a sign? In: Collected papers. Harvard University Press, Cambridge Mass., pp 1931-1935
5. De Saussure F (1916) Corso di linguistica generale [Course of general linguistics]. Laterza, Bari
6. Lakoff G (1987) Women, fire and dangerous thing: what categories reveal about the mind. Chicago University Press, Chicago
7. Giannoli GI (2005) La comprensione inferenziale. In: Ferretti F, Gambarara D (eds) Comunicazione e scienza cognitiva. Laterza, Bari, pp 73-110
8. Wittgenstein L (1953) Philosophische Untersuchungen. Blackwell, Oxford
9. Morris CW (1938) Foundations of the theory of signs. In: Neurath O, Carnap R, Morris CW (eds) International enciclopedy of unifies science. University of Chicago Press, Chicago, pp 77-138
10. Grice P (1975) Logic and conversation. In: Cole P, Morgan JL (eds) Syntax and semantics 3: Speech acts. Academic Press, New York, pp 41-58
11. Searle JR (1969) Speech acts: an essay in the philosophy of language. Cambridge University Press, Cambridge
12. Searle JR (1976) A classification of illocutionary acts. Language in Society 5:1-23
13. Verschueren J (1999) Understanding Pragmatics. Arnold, London
14. Ferretti F, Gambarara D (2005) Comunicazione e scienza cognitiva [Communication and cognitive science]. Laterza, Bari
15. Sperber D, Wilson D (1986) Relevance: communication and cognition. Blackwell, Oxford
16. Levinson S (2000) Presumptive meanings: the theory of generalized conversational implicature. The MIT Press, Cambridge, MA
17. Récanati F (2003) Literal meaning. Cambridge University Press, Cambridge
18. Carston R (2002) Thoughts and utterances: the pragmatics of explicit communication. Blackwell, Oxford
19. Sperber D, Noveck I (2004) Experimental pragmatics. Palgrave, San Diego

20. Giora R (2003) On our mind: context, salience and figurative language. Oxford University Press, New York
21. Gibbs RW (1999) Speakers' intuitions and pragmatic theory. Cognition 69:355-359
22. Gibbs RW (2002) A new look at literal meaning in understanding what is said and implicated. J Pragmatics 34:457-486
23. Stemmer B (1999) Pragmatics: theoretical and clinical issues. Brain Lang 68:389-391
24. Stemmer B, Shönle PW (2000) Neuropragmatics in the 21st century. Brain Lang 71:233-236
25. Stemmer B (2008) Neuropragmatics: disorders and neural systems. In: Stemmer B, Whitaker HA (eds) Handbook of the neuroscience of language. Elsevier, Amsterdam, pp 177-198
26. Hird K, Kirsner K (2003) The effect of right cerebral hemisphere damage on collaborative planning in conversation: an analysis of intentional structure. Clin Linguist Phonet 17:309-325
27. Joanette Y, Ansaldo AY (1999) Clinical note: acquired pragmatic impairments and aphasia. Brain Lang 68:529-534
28. McDonald S (1998) Communication and language disturbances following traumatic brain injury. In: Stemmer B, Whitaker HA (eds) Handbook of neurolinguistics. Academic, San Diego London, pp 485-494
29. Martin I, McDonald S (2003) Weak coherence, no theory of mind, or executive dysfunction? Solving the puzzle of pragmatic language disorders. Brain Lang 85:451-466
30. Kacinik NA, Chiarello C (2007) Understanding metaphors: is the right brain uniquely involved? Brain Lang 100:188-207
31. Mason RA, William DL, Kana RK et al (2008) Theory of mind disruption and recruitment of the right hemisphere during narrative comprehension in autism. Neuropsychologia 46:269-280
32. Giora R, Zaidel E, Soroker N et al (2000) Differential effects of right- and left-hemisphere damage on understanding sarcasm and metaphor. Metaphor Symbol 15:63-83
33. Noveck IA, Posada A (2003) Characterizing the time course of an implicature: an evoked potentials study. Brain Lang 85:203-210
34. Buchanan TW, Lutz K, Mirzazade S et al (2000) Recognition of emotional prosody and verbal components of spoken language: an fMRI study. Cognitive Brain Res 9:227-238
35. Lee SS, Dapretto M (2006) Metaphorical vs. literal word meanings: fMRI evidence against a selective role of the right hemisphere. Neuroimage 15:536-544
36. Coulson S (2004) Electrophysiology and pragmatic language comprehension. In: Sperber D, Noveck IA (eds) Experimental pragmatics. Palgrave, San Diego, pp 187-206
37. Keller J, Recht T (1998) Towards a modular description of the deficits in spontaneous speech in dementia. J Pragmatics 29:313-332
38. Kutas M (2006) One lesson learned: frame language processing – literal and figurative – as a human brain function. Metaphor Symbol 4:285-325
39. Caplan D (1992) Language: structure, processing and disorders. The MIT Press, Cambridge, MA
40. Joanette Y, Goulet P, Hannequin D (1990) Right hemisphere and verbal communication. Springer, New York
41. Beeman M, Chiarello C (1998) Right hemisphere language comprehension: perspectives from cognitive neuroscience. Erlbaum, Hillsdale, New Jersey
42. Zaidel E (1998) Language in the right hemisphere following callosal disconnection. In: Stemmer B, Whitaker HA (eds) Handbook of neurolinguistics. Academic, San Diego, pp 369-383
43. Kumon-Nakamura S, Glucksberg S, Brown M (1995) How about another piece of pie: the allusional pretense theory of discourse irony. J Experimental Psychol Gen 124:3-21
44. Attardo S (2000) Irony as relevant inappropriateness. J Pragmatics 32:793-826

5

45. Gibbs RW (1994) The poetics of mind: figurative thought and figurative language. Academic Press, San Diego
46. Kihara Y (2005) The mental space structure of verbal irony. Cognitive Linguist 16:513-530
47. Ritchie D (2005) Frame-shifting in humor and irony. Metaphor Symbol 20:275-294
48. Colston HL, O'Brien J (2000) Contrast and pragmatics in figurative language: anything understatement can do, irony can do better. J Pragmatics 32:1557-1583
49. Utsumi A (2000) Verbal irony as implicit display of ironic environment: distinguishing ironic utterances from nonirony. J Pragmatics 32:1777-1806
50. Giora R, Fein O, Schwartz T (1998) Irony: graded salience and indirect negation. Metaphor Symbol 13:83-101
51. Dews S, Winner E (1999) Obligatory processing of literal and nonliteral meanings in verbal irony. J Pragmatics 31:1579-1599
52. Gibbs RW (1999) Interpreting what speakers say and implicate. Brain Lang 68:466-485
53. Ivanko SL, Pexman PM (2003) Context incongruity and irony processing. Discourse Process 35:241-279
54. Long DL, Graesser AC (1988) Wit and humour in discourse processes. Discourse Process 11:35-60
55. Shamay-Tsoory SG, Tomer R, Ahron-Peretz J (2005) The neuroanatomical basis of understanding sarcasm and its relationship to social cognition. Neuropsychology 19:288-300
56. Colston HL, Katz AN (eds) (2005) Figurative language comprehension: social and cultural influences. Erlbaum, Hillsdale, New Jersey
57. Schwoebel J, Dews S, Winner E, Srinivas K (2000) Obligatory processing of the literal meaning of ironic utterances: further evidence. Metaphor Symbol 15:47-61
58. Balconi, M, Tutino, S (2007) An ERP analysis of iconic language and iconic thinking. The case of metaphor. J Int Neuropsych Soc 13, supplement 2:74
59. Coulson S, van Petten C (2002) Conceptual integration and metaphor: an event-related potential study. Mem Cognit 30:958-968
60. Pynte J, Besson M, Robichon FH, Poli J (1996) The time-course of metaphor comprehension: an event-related potential study. Brain Lang 55:293-316
61. Tartter VC, Gomes H, Dubrovsky B et al (2002) Novel metaphors appear anomalous at least momentarily: evidence from N400. Brain Lang 80:488-509
62. Cornejo C, Simonetti F, Aldunate N et al (2007) Electrophysiological evidences of different interpretative strategies in irony comprehension. J Psycholing Res 36:411-430
63. Balconi M, Amenta S (2007) Neuropsychological processes in verbal irony comprehension: an event-related potentials (ERPs) investigation. J Int Neuropsych Soc 13, Supplement 2:77
64. Balconi M, Amenta S (2009) Pragmatic and semantic information interplay in ironic meaning computation: Evidence from "pragmatic-semantic" P600 effect. J Int Neuropsychol Soc 15:86
65. McDonald S (1999) Exploring the process of inference generation in sarcasm: a review of normal and clinical studies. Brain Lang 68:486-506
66. McDonald S (2000) Neuropsychological studies on sarcasm. Metaphor and Symbol 15:85-98
67. Brownell HH, Simpson TL, Bihrle AM et al (1990) Appreciation of metaphoric alternative word meanings by left and right brain-damaged patients. Neuropsychologia 28:375-383
68. Winner E, Brownell H, Happe F et al (1998) Distinguishing lies from jokes: theory of mind deficits and discourse interpretation in right hemisphere brain-damaged patients. Brain Lang 62:89-106
69. Stuss DT, Gallup GG Jr, Alexander MP (2001) The frontal lobes are necessary for theory of mind. Brain 124:279-286
70. McDonald S, Pearce S (1996) Clinical insights into pragmatic theory: frontal lobe deficits and sarcasm. Brain Lang 53:81-104

71. Ross ED (2000) Affective prosody and the aprosodias. In: Mesulam MM (ed) Principles of behavioral and cognitive neurology. Oxford University Press, New York, pp 316-331
72. Uekermann J, Channon S, Winkel K et al (2007) Theory of mind, humour processing and executive functioning in alcoholism. Addiction 102:232-240
73. Romero Lauro LJ, Tettamanti M, Cappa SF, Papagno C (2008) Idiom comprehension: a prefrontal task? Cereb Cortex 18:162-170
74. Amanzio M, Geminiani G, Leotta D, Cappa S (2008) Metaphor comprehension in Alzheimer disease: novelty matters. Brain Lang 107:1-10
75. Pell MD (2007) Reduced sensitivity to prosodic attitudes in adults with focal right hemisphere brain damage. Brain Lang 101:64-79
76. Walker J, Fongemie K, Daigle T (2001) Prosodic facilitation in the resolution of syntactic ambiguities in subjects with left and right hemisphere damage. Brain Lang 78:169-196
77. Baum SR, Dwivedi VD (2003) Sensitivity to prosodic structure in left- and right-hemisphere-damaged individuals. Brain Lang 87:278-289
78. Tompkins CA, Mateer CA (1985) Right hemisphere appreciation of prosodic and linguistic indications of implicit attitude. Brain Lang 24:185–203
79. Eviatar Z, Just MA (2006) Brain correlates of discourse processing: an fMRI investigation of irony and conventional metaphors comprehension. Neuropsychologia 44:2348-2359
80. Uchiyama H, Seki A, Kageyama H et al (2006) Neural substrates of sarcasm: a functional magnetic-resonance imaging study. Brain Res 1124:100-110
81. Ting Wang A, Lee SS, Sigman M, Dapretto M (2006) Developmental changes in the neural basis of interpreting communicative intent. Scan 1:107-121
82. Caplan R, Dapretto M (2001) Making sense during conversation: an fMRI study. Neuroreport 12:3625-3632
83. Haxby JV, Hoffman EA, Gobbini MI (2002) Human neural systems for face recognition and social communication. Biol Psych 51:59-67

Idiomatic Language Comprehension: Neuropsychological Evidence

6

C. Papagno

6.1 Introduction

Idioms [1] are conventional expressions, in general deeply connected to culture, whose meaning cannot be derived from an analysis of the constituent words' typical meanings (e.g., to kick the bucket). *Conventionality* gives an idea of the strength of the association between an idiomatic expression and its meaning within a given culture and is determined by the discrepancy between the idiomatic phrasal meaning and the meaning we would predict for the collocation if we were to consult only the rules to determine the meanings of the constituents in isolation [2]. Idioms do not form a unitary class and rather vary along a number of syntactic and semantic dimensions [2, 3]. For example, they vary as to their semantic *transparency/opacity*, which refers to the ease with which the motivation for their structure can be recovered. Idioms can involve figuration and can be originally metaphorical (e.g., *take the bull by the horns*), even if speakers may not perceive the figure originally involved; in this specific example, a potentially dangerous situation is evoked, which is faced directly; in such a case, the idiom is called transparent. By contrast, an expression such as *farsene un baffo* (literal translation: *make oneself a moustache*, meaning to not care about something) is semantically opaque, since the speaker needs to know the stipulated meaning, which cannot be derived either from the image evoked or from the constituent word meanings. Opaque expressions are also based on a historical or cultural motivation, but in most cases, this has since been forgotten or cannot be directly perceived by the speaker [4]. Idioms vary as to their *decomposability*, meaning the extent to which the idiomatic interpretation can be mapped onto single constituents [5]. For example, in *to empty the sack*, the verb *to empty* directly suggests the action

C. Papagno (✉)
Department of Psychology, University of Milano-Bicocca, Milan, Italy

6

of *taking out*, i.e., to reveal, while the term *sack* evokes a container; in other cases, however, the idiomatic interpretation cannot be mapped onto the single constituents, such as in *kick the bucket*. Although there may be some relation between the two notions (decomposability and transparency), they do not overlap. While some idioms, like *spill the beans*, may be decomposable and opaque, others may be non-decomposable and transparent. For example, *saw logs* has no identifiable parts mapping onto the meaning; yet, the acoustic communalities between a saw cutting wood and the noise made by some sleepers is not hard to appreciate. Idioms vary in the extent to which they can be syntactically transformed while still retaining their idiomatic meaning [6]. They typically occur only in limited syntactic constructions, even though there is a large variability among them, and while some are almost completely unconstrained (e.g., *spill the beans*, *let the cat out of the bag*), others allow very few operations, if any (e.g., *by and large*). This depends on the degree of their *syntactic frozenness*. Finally, many idioms (known as "ambiguous" idioms) can also be assigned a literal interpretation (e.g., *break the ice*), while others do not have any well-formed literal counterpart (for example, in Italian, *far venire il latte alle ginocchia*, whose literal translation is *to make the milk come up to one's knees*, means to be extremely boring) and are unambiguous [7, 8]. The exact role of these characteristics is still an open question, but there is little doubt that they can affect comprehension.

Recently, an increasing number of studies have investigated figurative language in brain-damaged patients [9-13]. In most of them, group studies were performed using comprehension tasks with the aim of investigating hemispheric lateralization. However, a common limit of neuropsychological studies is to consider all the different forms of figurative language as a single class. In particular, in the case of metaphors and idioms it is not unusual to find idioms that have been considered as if they were metaphors, and vice versa. In addition, when only idiomatic expressions are studied, no distinction is made along the parameters described above (transparency, decomposability, syntactic frozenness, ambiguity).

Idiom comprehension has been investigated in different pathological populations, such as in focal brain-damaged patients, patients with Alzheimer's disease (AD), and schizophrenic patients. Recently, electrophysiological techniques have been employed as well, such as repetitive transcranial magnetic stimulation (rTMS) and event-related potentials (ERP), but also neuroimaging procedures, in particular functional magnetic resonance (fMRI).

In this chapter, I will not discuss idiom production, since, to date, experimental and clinical studies on brain-damaged patients specifically devoted to this topic are lacking. Typically, aphasic patients automatically produce familiar phrases, including idioms, which are expressed with a normal prosody and well-articulated. Traditionally, the spared production of familiar phrases is attributed to the language capacity of the right hemisphere.

6.2 Experimental Paradigms

Idiom comprehension in patients with focal brain damage has been investigated by means of many different paradigms, with the consequence of making comparisons among studies almost impossible. Most of these paradigms involved off-line measurements. The most popular approach, easily carried out in aphasic patients, is a sentence-to-picture matching task. The patient is presented with a sentence, either by auditory or visual means, and has to select the picture that corresponds most closely to the sentence, choosing between two, three, or four options. This modality has a crucial limitation: indeed, there is no univocal representation of a figurative expression in general and of an idiom in particular, so that a subject can refuse the target simply because it does not satisfy his/her personal idea of how to represent it. Other possible paradigms examine lexical decision, reaction times, and sentence reading. In lexical decision, patients hear or read several priming sentences and then perform a lexical decision task on target stimuli (words and non-words). Priming sentences can be idiomatic or literal, and target words can be related to either the idiomatic or the literal meaning. When reaction times are evaluated, patients hear a sentence including a specified target word and the task is to press a key as soon as the target word appears. In this case, sentences are of three different types: idiomatic, literal (the same sentences are used, but the context can suggest one or another interpretation), and control sentences. Less frequently, an oral definition of idiomatic expressions or a sentence-to-word association in a four-choice condition is required. Idiomatic expressions should be carefully selected, taking into account all the relevant variables such as familiarity (to what extent an idiom is known among a specific population), transparency, and ambiguity. Recently, ambiguous and unambiguous idioms were investigated in separate studies, as well as verbal and nominal idiomatic phrases.

6.3 Idiom Comprehension in Patients with Focal Brain Lesions

6.3.1 Idiom Comprehension in Right-brain-damaged Patients

A widely accepted view in the earliest neuropsychological literature on idiom comprehension assumed that damage to the left hemisphere had no major consequences; rather, it is the non-dominant right hemisphere that is important for the processing of idiomatic expressions (see [14] for a review). This hypothesis was based on a misinterpretation of the first reported study on figurative language [15]. Winner and Gardner, indeed, found that aphasic left-brain-damaged (LBD) patients correctly associated metaphoric expressions with the corresponding picture, whereas right-brain-damaged (RBD) patients, despite being able to give correct verbal explanations, chose the picture corresponding to the literal meaning. By contrast, the five LBD patients of that study, who were tested in the oral modality, gave a literal explanation despite choosing the metaphorical picture. Although this finding has been taken as evidence that RBD patients are impaired in figurative language, it may only indicate that RBD patients are defective in picture matching. Accordingly, a greater difficulty with pictorial material is constantly reported when RBD patients are tested. In addition, only metaphors were used and the results cannot be generalized to other forms of figurative language. In the same year, Stachowiak et al. [16] investigated semantic and pragmatic strategies in the comprehension of spoken texts in four subgroups of aphasic patients and in normal and RBD patients. Short texts of similar linguistic structure were read to the subjects, who were required to choose the picture that was appropriate to the story from a multiple choice set of five. Besides a picture showing the main event of the story, one picture depicted the literal sense of a metaphorical comment, while the others misrepresented semantic functions (subject noun phrase, verb, verb complement phrase) expressed in the text. For example, in a story about an office employee getting himself involved in too much work, the idiomatic comment was *he got himself into a nice mess* (literally from German: *he filled his soup with pieces of bread*). Half of the stories were commented with transparent (close relationship between metaphorical and literal sense) idioms and half with opaque (remote relationship) idioms. Apparently, performance was better for opaque idioms and in general the groups did not differ. However, Wernicke's aphasics showed particular difficulties in dealing with metaphorical (transparent) idioms, pointing to the literal interpretation.

A very influential paper and a later similar one [17, 18] reported a double dissociation between idiom comprehension and novel sentence comprehension in LBD and RBD patients: while RBD participants had a normal performance with novel (literal) sentences and a poor one with familiar (figurative) sentences, aphasic patients showed the opposite pattern. However, several criticisms could be applied to the approach used in these studies. First, even if the literal and non-literal sentences were matched in structure, items were not chosen on the basis of their intrinsic linguistic features (transparency/opacity, decomposability, etc.), and idioms, proverbs, and courtesy phrases were considered together as "familiar language." Second, the number of stimuli was limited. Third, clinical features, such as the severity of aphasia and the modalities of assessment, were not always described; other neuropsychological (attentional, perceptual, spatial) deficits were not tested (or the test results not reported). This last point is especially relevant since when sensory or cognitive deficits associated with right hemisphere damage result in suboptimal processing of critical elements or deplete available resources needed for further analysis, patients might be particularly likely to resort to the less demanding choice (the literal alternative, which exactly corresponds to the sentence) in a sentence-to-picture matching task. Visuo-perceptual and visuo-spatial abilities are more relevant for pictures representing idiomatic meanings, as picture complexity is higher for idiomatic than for literal sentences. Literal sentences allow a single interpretation, and limited visuo-spatial and attentional resources could still be sufficient in this case, but not when an abstract meaning is to be depicted. Studies of RBD patients with neglect, showing a significant correlation between performance on an idiom comprehension task (using a sentence-to-picture matching paradigm) and star cancellation and line bisection accuracy, support this hypothesis [19]. Finally, in the study of Van Lancker and Kempler [17], the performance of aphasic patients was considered to be normal for familiar phrases, but the mean percentage of correct responses was 72%, while that of control subjects was 97.3%. However, Van Lancker and Kempler were the first to create a standardized test, the Familiar and Novel Language Comprehension Test (FANL-C), which was developed to avoid verbal output and to limit metalinguistic functioning. The patient is shown a set of four line drawings and asked to select the one that matches a sentence read aloud by the examiner. There are 40 test items, comprising 20 familiar phrases, including proverbs, idioms, and contextually bound social interaction formulas (*I'll get back to you later*), and 20 novel sentences constructed to match the familiar ones in length, surface grammatical structure, and word frequency. The foils for familiar phrases include two concrete interpretations that are related to individual words in the stimulus sentence (the picture is described by a sentence containing a content word of the familiar phrase); the third foil represents the opposite figurative meaning of the familiar phrase. There is no depiction of a correct literal interpretation (in contrast with a previous version of the test by the same authors), since, in the authors' view, this could also be considered correct. Two sample items are used to demonstrate the task prior to administering the test items. Responses and time required to complete each subtest are reported on the protocol. Performance is evaluated as the total number of correct responses and total time needed to accomplish each subtest. Mean scores and standard deviations from a sample of 335 neurologically unimpaired subjects, ranging from age 3 to age 80 years were reported; however, the level of education was not considered, although this is relevant for idioms.

The problem concerning the implications of the nature and use of idiom interpretation tasks was raised by Tompkins et al. [20]. Indeed, they correctly argued that defining an idiomatic phrase or choosing a pictured representation is the end product of multiple aspects of mental work, so the source of failure on such tasks is not clear. In other words, off-line tasks are distant in time (and correspondingly in terms of cognitive operations) from the initial retrieval or computation of meaning. By contrast, on-line tasks require a response to some aspect of the input during, rather than after, the comprehension process. In order to verify the possibility of obtaining different results depending on the type of task (off-line *vs* on-line), Tompkins et al. tested 20 RBD patients (40% of them showing signs of neglect), 20 with LBD (65% of them being aphasic), and 20 control subjects without known neurological impairment. Participants performed two tasks of idiom comprehension. The primary task was an on-line word-monitoring task in which subjects listened for a specified target word in a spoken sentence and pressed a button as quickly as possible when they heard it. Target words (e.g., *rat*) were concrete nouns that were the final elements of ambiguous familiar phrases (e.g., *smell a rat*). Response times were recorded for target monitoring in three experimental context conditions: idiomatic, literal, and control. Contexts consisted of two sentences, with the target noun embedded in the second: idiomatic and literal contexts contained the target noun in its familiar idiomatic phrase (e.g., *smelled a rat*) but forced the interpretation of the phrase to be non-literal or literal, respectively. In control contexts, the target noun did not occur in a familiar phrase (e.g., saw a rat). Finally, filler contexts were created for each target word and were similar in structure and complexity to the idiomatic and literal contexts. Brain-damaged subjects performed similarly to normal controls on this task; all three groups responded more quickly to target nouns in idiomatic phrases (in either idiomatic or literal biasing contexts). In the off-line task, 12 highly familiar idiomatic phrases were selected, and participants were required to give a definition of each. In this task, brain-damaged subjects fared poorly, making more errors than controls, with no difference between RBD and LBD. Therefore, adults with unilateral brain damage seem to be able to activate and retrieve familiar idiomatic forms and their idiom interpretation deficits most likely reflect impairment at some later stage of information processing. However, two points should be noted. First, only 65% of LBD patients were aphasic and one could argue that aphasic patients, if considered separately, would have been found impaired on the on-line task. In addition, no information about the lesion site or size was given, only a rough distinction among anterior, posterior, mixed, and subcortical lesions. Second, ambiguous idioms were tested, and aphasic patients seem to show more severe deficits with unambiguous idioms (see below).

6.3.2
Idiom Comprehension in Aphasic Patients

More recently, the right hemisphere hypothesis has been challenged and neuropsychological studies have emphasized the involvement of the left hemisphere, specifically the temporal lobe, in idiom comprehension. Indeed, in a sentence-to-picture matching task using three alternatives (one picture representing the idiomatic interpretation, one representing as well as possible the literal interpretation, one representing an unrelated situation), aphasic (both fluent and non-fluent) patients proved to be severely impaired. Idioms were highly familiar, opaque, and unambiguous (in that the literal meaning was implausible or the sentence was ill-formed). In patients who were able to give an oral definition of the items despite aphasia, performance increased but still remained significantly worse than that of controls. Idiom definition, however, cannot be administered to all patients, since their deficits may prevent an oral response. In addition, the picture-matching paradigm may lead to underestimation of the patient's ability to comprehend idiomatic expressions. The analysis of individual errors in the sentence-to-picture matching task showed that patients did not choose at random, as they selected the unrelated alternative only few times, producing a number of these errors that was entirely comparable with that of the healthy participants. A further analysis of responses given by aphasic patients with semantic deficits showed that they took advantage of syntactic information. In other words, presented with ill-formed idioms, for example, *tenere banco*, literally *to hold bench*, in which the syntactically correct (but not idiomatically correct) Italian form would be *tenere il banco*, patients with good syntactic competence made fewer literal errors than with well-formed idioms; these patients engaged in the retrieval of the figurative interpretation only when the linguistic analysis of the string failed to yield acceptable results. Therefore, aphasic patients make use of spared language abilities in order to comprehend idiomatic expressions: syntactic competence [12] when lexical-semantic knowledge is impaired, and semantic knowledge when syntactic analysis is defective [11]. When syntactic competence is spared and semantic knowledge is impaired, aphasic patients accept the literal interpretation of well-formed idioms, even when this is implausible; since they show semantic deficits, they do not recognize that the sentence is implausible.

In patients with syntactic deficits but spared semantic knowledge [11], performance was found to correlate with the plausibility of the literal interpretation: the more plausible the literal interpretation, the greater the probability that the patient will select this picture when presented with the idiomatic expression. When LBD and RBD patients are compared, aphasic patients are significantly impaired not only relative to matched controls, but also to RBD patients [19]. These findings are consistent with the view that idioms are subject to processes very similar to those involved in the comprehension of literal expressions; in particular, they undergo a full syntactic analysis. These results cannot be explained within the lexical hypothesis [21], according to which idioms are mentally represented and recognized as long, morphologically complex words that do not undergo syntactic analysis. These data also counter any idiom comprehension model based on mental imagery: when faced with idioms, it is possible to resort to at least two sources of meaning, literal and figurative. The results of the picture-matching paradigm show that whenever an image is selected by a brain-damaged patient to represent an idiomatic sentence, it definitely does not correspond to the figurative meaning [3].

As already stated, idiomatic expressions are not a homogeneous class. Typically, opaque non-ambiguous idioms were used in studies with aphasic patients. Yet, it is possible that different types of expression undergo different types of processing. Information is available also for ambiguous idioms, namely, expressions for which the literal meaning is plausible [22]. In this case, a different testing modality, the word-to-sentence matching task, has been used more frequently. Syntactically simple sentences paired with four words are presented and the task is to choose the one that corresponds to the figurative meaning. The four words are matched in terms of length and written frequency: the target word corresponds to the idiomatic interpretation of the string (e.g., *wine*, for *alzare il gomito*, literally *to raise the elbow*, meaning to drink too much); one foil is semantically associated with the last constituent word of the idiom string (in the previous example, *leg*); and two words are unrelated foils (*tree*, *box*) (Fig. 6.1). Specifically, the first type of unrelated target is either an abstract or a concrete word depending on the nature of the idiomatic target: the unrelated target is abstract if the idiomatic target is abstract, and concrete if the idiomatic target is concrete. A target word is considered as concrete based on the availability of the word referent to sensory experience. The second type of unrelated target is a word that could plausibly complete the verb in the verb phrase (*box*). The rationale underlying the selection of these four types of targets was the following: the choice

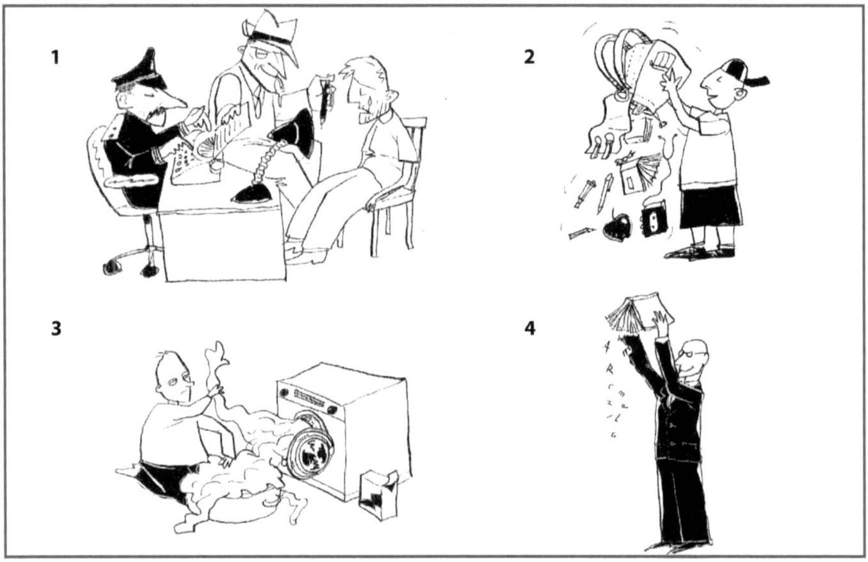

Fig. 6.1 Examples of alternatives for the expression, translated from the Italian as *to empty the sack* (meaning *to confess something*). **1** Figurative target; **2** semantically associated foil: the last word of the sentence describing this picture is of the same semantic category as the last word of the target sentence; **3** the verb is followed by a congruent noun; **4** the last word of the sentence describing this picture is concrete as the last word of the target sentence

of the idiomatic target should reflect the knowledge and availability of the idiomatic meaning of the idiom string. The choice of the semantically associated foil might reflect an attempt at interpreting the string literally when the patient does not know the idiom meaning; alternatively, she/he may be unable to access the idiomatic interpretation of the idiom string. The semantic associate foil, however, does not reflect the literal meaning of the sentence and its choice is clearly an error. The two unrelated foils should signal an impaired performance of both the idiomatic and the literal processing of the string.

Aphasic patients were significantly more impaired in idiom comprehension than matched controls, even with this different type (ambiguous) of expression. Semantic-associate errors were indeed significantly more frequent than unrelated errors. Two explanations might be provided for the high level of selection of semantically associated foils: the first relies on the idea that no access to the corresponding figurative meaning can occur without identification of the idiomatic nature of the string. In aphasic patients what might be deficient is the idiom recognition mechanism. Alternatively, one can hypothesize that semantically associated errors reflect impairment in inhibiting the word meaning associated with the final constituent word of the idiom string or a faster activation of that meaning. If this were the case, then the retrieval of the figurative meaning would be blocked by a sort of processing loop in which the patient is unable to get rid of the literal meaning of the string. It could also be possible that the choice of the semantically related target only reflects a lexical association with the last word of the string, without a global processing at a sentential level. However, previous evidence on the comprehension of idioms in brain-damaged patients suggests that their impairment extends far beyond the single-word level.

In general, however, patients tend to choose the literal response, in both the sentence-to-picture matching and the sentence-to-word matching task. Eventually, since language resources are damaged in aphasics, a greater involvement of executive control is required in linguistic tasks, thus depleting the attentional pool and preventing the appropriate suppression/inhibition of the literal meaning, even when it is less salient than the figurative one.

As reported, off-line tasks were employed in the experiments described above although we do not know for sure what they measure. Converging evidence, using different tasks and methodologies, could strengthen and clarify the results. Along this line, 15 aphasic patients were submitted to three tasks of unambiguous idiom comprehension: a sentence-to-picture matching task, a sentence-to-word matching task, and an oral definition task. A high variability emerged among the aphasic patients; some of them were severely impaired, while others performed at parity with the control group [23]. The performance was not exclusively related to the severity of the language deficit in general, except in the case of oral definition, which could not be accomplished in severe non-fluent patients. Several factors appear to play a role, apart from lexical semantic and syntactic abilities. The type of task had a relevant effect on the patients' performance, but not on that of healthy subjects. The overt representation of the literal meaning, namely a bizarre picture corresponding to some form of literal interpretation, had a strong interference effect, similar to the Stroop effect. Patients are unable to suppress the literal interpretation when its explicit pictorial representation is available; this suggests that the literal interpretation somehow remains active while the sentence is being processed, even when it has a very low plausibility. In the sentence-to-picture matching task, patients and controls very rarely choose the picture corresponding to the "single word" option. For example, in the case of the Italian idiom translated as *to come to the hand*, meaning *to fight*. The single word option would be a picture representing a boy lifting his hand (Fig. 6.2). This type of error occurred with the same frequency as the unrelated error type, suggesting that some level of processing of the sentential literal meaning took place and that the patients' choice was not only influenced by a lexical effect.

The sentence-to-word matching task, with no literal alternatives but with a semantic foil (in the previous example *finger*), reduces the interference of the literal interpretation of the string with unambiguous idioms, but unrelated errors are still present and seem to indicate a lack of knowledge of the idiomatic meaning. Since literal errors appeared especially when the literal interpretation was overtly "offered" to the patient, it could be possible that the figurative meaning was lost (or not accessed) and, when the literal alternative was not present, an unrelated error, preserving the semantic class (abstract/concrete), was produced. This is a further demonstration that the patient tries to analyze the whole sentence and does not process a single word only. The different pattern of errors produced with unambigu-

6

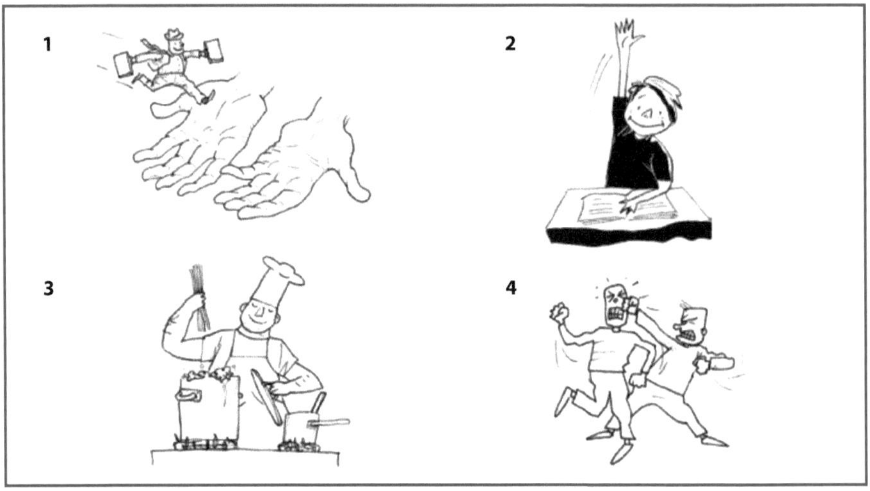

Fig. 6.2 Examples of alternatives for the non-ambiguous expression, translated from the Italian as, *to come to the hands* (meaning *to fight*). **1** literal foil; **2** single-word foil; **3** unrelated foil; **4** idiomatic target

ous and ambiguous idioms in the sentence-to-word paradigm (significantly more unrelated errors preserving the semantic class, and significantly more literal associate errors, respectively) suggests a different type of processing. Additional support for this hypothesis is provided by the double dissociation observed in aphasic patients: while some patients are severely impaired on ambiguous idiom comprehension and give a noticeably better performance on unambiguous idioms, other patients make no errors on ambiguous idioms and perform at chance on unambiguous idioms. Overall, aphasic patients unexpectedly showed a better performance with ambiguous idioms, as if a plausible literal meaning helped in retrieving the idiomatic one: this result deserves further investigation.

A different paradigm, showing that not all idiomatic expressions are processed alike, was used with a deep dyslexic patient. The reading of Finnish verb-phrase idioms was compared with that of noun-phrase idioms [10]: on the basis of a series of experiments, it was concluded that noun-phrase idioms are processed more holistically than verb-phrase idioms, which were processed in the same way as control literal sentences. The verb-phrase idioms were read as poorly as comparable free phrases and morphological errors at the verb were produced. Noun-phrase idioms were easier for the patient who produced errors in noun phrases that contained inflected nouns.

Although there is evidence of impairment of idiomatic processing in aphasia, aphasic patients with a normal performance have also been described [24], as was the case of two German LBD patients, one with Wernicke's aphasia and the other with global aphasia, in a cross-modal lexical priming paradigm. This result, however, does not contradict previously reported findings, since stimuli were German noun compounds, which can have both idiomatic and literal meanings. Indeed, noun-phrase idioms have proved to be easier to access than verb-phrase idioms, which were indeed the most frequent form of idiomatic expressions used in previously reported studies.

From an anatomical point of view, a general analysis of the relevant lesions shows that two sites are involved in patients' performance on idiom comprehension: a cortical and/or subcortical frontal area, which seems particularly involved in the case of ambiguous idioms, and a cortical temporal region, which is constantly damaged when unambiguous idiom comprehension is impaired. These results are supported by several rTMS experiments using off-line [25] and on-line [26, 27] paradigms and a sentence-to-picture matching task. Left temporal rTMS (off-line) applied over BA22 increased reaction times and reduced accuracy, without significant differences between idiomatic and literal sentences. In a study that explored the temporal dynamics of left prefrontal and temporal cortex in idiom processing by using on-line rTMS in normal subjects, a selective decrease in accuracy was found for idioms when rTMS was applied to the prefrontal (BA9) and temporal (BA22) cortex 80 ms after picture presentation, confirming the role of these regions in the task. Moreover, rTMS to the prefrontal cortex, but not to the temporal cortex, continued to affect the performance with idiomatic sentences at a later time of 120 ms. These results suggest that the prefrontal region is involved in both the retrieval of the figurative meaning from semantic memory and the monitoring of the response by inhibiting alternative interpretations [26].

6.3.3 Idiom Comprehension and the Prefrontal Lobe

Based on the above discussion, it is clear that in idiom interpretation both linguistic and non-linguistic processes are called into account. Support for this view comes from a study on a patient diagnosed with Down's syndrome [28]. Some aspects of her executive functions were severely impaired, but propositional language was normal. Accordingly, RBD patients seem to be impaired only when the lesion is localized in the prefrontal (cortical or subcortical) region; otherwise the performance of RBD patients is not different from that of neurologically unimpaired subjects. Patients with a right prefrontal lesion perform as badly as aphasic patients with a temporal lesion. These data have been confirmed by rTMS experiments. Besides the previously noted chronometric study, both right and left BA9 stimulation [27] reduced reaction times and increased the number of errors in an idiom comprehension task (sentence-to-picture paradigm). A faster response with less accuracy suggests a release from inhibition. The finding of a role of the right (and not only the left) dorsolateral prefrontal cortex (but also of the subcortical white matter) could explain why figurative (and idiomatic, in particular) language impairment has been considered a consequence of RBD: since the exact lesion site is not reported in these studies, it could well be the case that a number of patients had a prefrontal lesion.

A bilateral prefrontal involvement in idiom processing is confirmed also by fMRI activation studies that have used different paradigms, such as deciding whether or not

6

the meaning of a sentence, either literal or idiomatic, matches a picture [29], or whether or not a word is related with a previously visually presented (either idiomatic or literal) sentence [30]. The results revealed that making judgments about literal and non-literal sentences yields a common network of cortical activity, involving language areas of the left hemisphere. However, the non-literal task elicited overall greater activation, in terms of magnitude and of spatial extent. Activation of the temporal cortex was also found, as predicted by neuropsychological and rTMS studies. In addition, the left superior frontal (approximately covering BA9) and left inferior frontal gyri were specifically involved in processing idiomatic sentences. Activations were also seen in the right superior and middle temporal gyri, in the temporal pole, and in the right inferior frontal gyrus. Recently, involvement of the medial superior frontal gyrus in idiom comprehension was confirmed using a different paradigm (inserting the idioms in short sentences, auditorily presented) [31].

Frontal regions could be involved for two reasons. Firstly, once the sentence is linguistically analyzed, producing two possible interpretations, the literal and the figurative, a response must be chosen. This requires a selection process and response monitoring; selection and monitoring of internally generated responses are likely to be performed by the central executive, whose neural correlates are thought to be in the prefrontal lobe. Indeed, patients with prefrontal lesions produce a higher number of literal interpretations than patients with non-frontal lesions. Secondly, the role of the prefrontal cortex in language control has been demonstrated in a number of activation studies, such as with tasks requiring sentence processing, in which the listener (or the reader) needs to maintain the information on-line for a given period.

6.3.4 Idiom Comprehension and the Corpus Callosum

It is evident that there is not a right hemispheric prevalence in idiom comprehension and a strict dichotomy is to be avoided; understanding idiomatic expressions requires at the very least all the lexical and extra-lexical skills involved in the understanding of literal discourse. In other words, idiomatic language follows the same procedure as literal language, plus a selection process between alternative meanings, which is likely to be supported by the inferior frontal gyrus, and a supplementary high-level cognitive process, supported by the anterior prefrontal cortex, possibly monitoring and integrating the results of the linguistic analysis and of the selection between competing meanings. Since both hemispheres are involved in complex processing, it is likely that the corpus callosum is also implicated. Idiom comprehension has been studied in children with spina bifida and agenesis and hypoplasia of the corpus callosum [32] by means of a sentence-to-picture matching task using idiomatic expressions, which were controlled for ambiguity and compositionality. Children with this anomaly were impaired with respect to non-decomposable idioms (idioms in which the literal meanings of the parts do not contribute to the overall literal interpretation and therefore linguistic context is more important than in decomposable idioms), showing slower reaction times and less accuracy than observed in age-matched children. The corpus callosum could be relevant in conflict resolution between two alternative meanings, the figurative and the idiomatic, at the end of which one is rejected; support for this theory comes from the fact that subjects with corpus callosum agenesis are more impaired when the literal meaning is particularly strong: when interhemispheric information transfer is degraded or at least slower, access to the figurative meaning could be more difficult. The difficulties particularly concern non-decomposable expressions, which require a stronger interhemispheric integration with contextual information.

6.4 Idiom Comprehension in Patients with Alzheimer's Disease

Inhibition/suppression of the literal meaning seems necessary for the correct interpretation of idioms. This function, as repeatedly emphasized, is attributed to the right and left prefrontal cortices, which are interconnected through the corpus callosum. The prefrontal cortex is an associative cortex and associative cortices become atrophic during neurodegenerative diseases, even if in AD the prefrontal involvement appears later on.

Language in AD patients has been extensively studied and verbal communication disorders are described as very frequent and early. AD patients are impaired in spontaneous speech, with prominent disturbances of semantics, while phonematic structures are preserved; figurative language is also impaired. Kempler, Van Lancker, and Read [33] examined 29 patients with probable AD ranging from mild (Mini Mental State Examination, MMSE score 28) to severe (MMSE score 2); they tested for word, idiom, and proverb (overall ten stimuli) and novel-phrase comprehension. In the figurative language comprehension task, no alternative corresponding to the literal interpretation was available, but only a referential representation of one word in the stimulus (concrete response). The results showed that AD patients had difficulty in interpreting abstract meanings: when faced with alternative interpretations of familiar phrases, they chose concrete responses, suggesting that they were using lexical (single-word), referential meaning to interpret the phrases. However, the variable degree of dementia (some patient had a MMSE score of 2) prevents any sensible conclusion.

A more recent study [34] investigated the impairment of figurative language comprehension in 39 patients with probable early AD; their score, on the Milan Overall Dementia Assessment (MODA), ranged between 62 and 80 (which corresponds to a MMSE score of 17–21). A verbal explanation of 20 nominal metaphors and 20 idiomatic sentences of different type (opaque/transparent, ambiguous/unambiguous) was required. The results showed that the decline of figurative language is not an early sign of dementia. A follow-up of 6–8 months in 23 patients did not show a significant impairment, especially when compared to literal language, which had severely worsened: verbal fluency on semantic cue and the Token Test were considered for production and comprehension assessment, respectively. This evolution suggests that the two aspects (figurative and literal) of language are somewhat independent. Indeed, 11 patients showed a double dissociation between figurative and literal language. However, only the extreme values were considered as dissociated, i.e., those cases with an equivalent score of 0 in one test and 3 and 4 in the other. Equivalent scores allow the performance obtained in one test to be compared with that obtained in other tests, which are standardized following the same procedure, once the confounding and potentially different effects of demographic variables have been removed [35]. This was done since we do not know the exact distribution in normal subjects of the differences between the original scores in the test. Therefore, a no-decision area was left, to make sure that only valid double dissociations would be included. Even with this constraint, eight patients were still left showing a double dissociation: six had an impairment of propositional (literal) language only, and two showed the opposite pattern, namely, an impairment of metaphor and idiom comprehension. This double dissociation rules out the possibility that metaphor and idiom comprehension is simply an easier task than the Token Test. There are two additional important results, which demonstrate how inappropriate it is to use metaphors and idioms as if they were identical parts of figurative language: first, one patient with a "strong" dissociation had normal metaphor comprehension and impaired idiom interpretation; second, the metaphors and idioms differed as far as the predominant kind of error was considered. While for idioms, the literal interpretation was the most frequent error, for metaphors an attempt was made to search for a figurative meaning, but this proved to be only partial or incorrect.

From an anatomical point of view, studies on AD patients are not particularly informative, but indirectly they confirm that figurative language comprehension depends, at least in part, on the integrity of the prefrontal cortex, which is impaired in a later stage of the disease. However, a deficit emerged in patients with early-stage AD when a sentence-to-picture paradigm and a specific category of idioms, namely unambiguous, were used [36]. In that study, 15 patients with mild probable AD had to choose between two pictures, one representing the figurative and the other the literal interpretation (implausible and represented by a bizarre picture). Patients were also submitted to a pencil-and-paper dual task, in order to evaluate executive functions, and to a literal sentence comprehension test. Whereas literal comprehension was normal in seven patients and mildly impaired in the others, idiom comprehension was very poor in all 15 patients compared to age- and education-matched controls and correlated with performance on the dual task. When the idiom test was repeated using an unrelated situation as an alternative to the picture representing the figurative meaning, performance significantly improved. This result suggests that the literal interpretation needs to be suppressed, but AD patients are unable to do so, although they have not lost the idiomatic meaning, as shown by the fact that they choose the correct answer when no literal representation is available. When the same patients are required to produce an oral explanation of the sentences, again some literal interpretation is produced whenever this represents a possible situation in the real world.

A similar impairment is also found in AD patients with respect to ambiguous idioms [37]. Fifteen AD patients were submitted to two tasks: a string-to-picture matching task and a string-to-word matching task. In the first, patients had to choose among four pictures, while in the second they had to choose among four words. For both tasks, the alternatives were the picture/word corresponding to the figurative meaning, a semantic associate (picture/word) to the last word of the idiom, and two unrelated alternatives, which were, in the case of words, an unrelated foil preserving the semantic class and a literal continuation foil (a word that can follow the verb in that sentence), while in the case of pictures the first alternative was substituted by an unrealistic foil. Idiom comprehension was poor and correlated with executive tasks: the dual task correlated with the sentence-to-word test and the Stroop test with the number of semantically related errors, which were the most frequent type of error produced (i.e., the longer the time needed to perform the Stroop test, the greater the number of semantic errors produced). Finally, correlation of the sentence-to-picture with the word-to-picture matching task was dramatically different between the two groups. While in the case of controls it proved to be significant, this was not the case for the AD patients. It is possible that, since AD patients are impaired in different cognitive domains, and, since tests are multifactorial, the result is an asymmetric, albeit pathological, performance in the two idiom tasks.

Schizophrenics' performance is particularly poor in the case of ambiguous idioms and the best predictors of performance proved to be the Wisconsin Card Sorting Test and a working memory task. Thought disorganization and cognitive decline did not appear to predict performance [41].

6.5 Idiom Comprehension in Schizophrenic Patients

Schizophrenic patients exhibit several neuropsychological deficits, which are described in 85% of that population and are considered a central component of the disease. Several different cognitive profiles have been reported: alternatively frontal lobe dysfunction, temporal lobe dysfunction, right hemisphere or left hemisphere involvement, and basal ganglia dysfunction. The hypothesis of a dysexecutive syndrome in schizophrenic patients has received particular attention. Indeed, schizophrenics perform poorly in executive tasks when the inhibition of irrelevant information, monitoring of incoming environmental stimuli, or coordination of tasks is required. Accordingly, the dorsolateral prefrontal cortex shows a significant degree of atrophy in morphological studies. Schizophrenic patients fail to adopt an abstract attitude; it is therefore reasonable to hypothesize that figurative language comprehension in general and idiom comprehension in particular should be impaired. Ambiguous idioms are the most severely impaired: when schizophrenic patients listened to sentences containing literally plausible and implausible idioms and made lexical decisions about idiom-related or literal-related targets, reduced priming for literally plausible idioms was found. By contrast, compared to controls, they showed intact priming for literally implausible idioms. This result suggests that schizophrenic patients make normal use of context to facilitate the activation of contextually appropriate meanings and are able to appreciate the relationship between context and subsequently encountered words. However, they are less able than controls to inhibit activation of contextually inappropriate material and are thus impaired when there is a need to select between two plausible interpretations. This dissociation in idiom priming effect suggests that a failure in abstract attitude does not globally affect all linguistic aspects [38]. Similar results were obtained using a task like the one adopted with aphasic patients to study ambiguous idiom comprehension. The idioms were presented untransformed and without any context, and every idiom was associated with four words, which referred to: (i) literal meaning, (ii) figurative meaning, (iii) concrete meaning (a word semantically related to the last word of the idiomatic sentence), (iv) inappropriate response (a word completely unrelated to the target) [39]. Even if the most frequently selected answer was the figurative alternative, schizophrenic patients chose a number of literal and concrete responses, which were absent in the case of participants without psychiatric deficits. However, these concrete responses are different from so-called concretistic thinking, since they do not refer to a concrete global interpretation of the idiom, but only to a single word of the idiom. Concrete responses in this task refer to the patient's tendency to focus on details before (and without) attempting the global meaning of the idioms. Recently, idiom comprehension was shown to be impaired in schizophrenics, by means of the oral definition task used with AD patients [35]. Since the score negatively correlated with the total error score in syntactic comprehension, it suggested that the processing of idioms involves not only pragmatic inference in the choice between two alternative meanings of an expression, but also syntactic abilities [40].

6.6 Conclusions

In conclusion, the main points that have emerged from the study of idiomatic expression comprehension in patients with neurological or psychiatric diseases are the following:

1. Rather than strict lateralization, a widely distributed network involving both hemispheres contributes to idiomatic processing. However, the role of the left temporal lobe is crucial for the initial analysis of the idiom meaning. Then, the bilateral prefrontal cortex is required to inhibit the less salient meaning of the sentence, namely, the literal one. Since both hemispheres are involved at this stage, as shown by neuropsychological, TMS, and fMRI studies, a lesion of the corpus callosum, the structure normally allowing interhemispheric transfer of information, can prevent a normal idiomatic processing.
2. Whilst task type has no influence on the performance of neurologically unimpaired participants, it does affect aphasic patients for a variety of reasons: reduced expressive skills in the case of oral definition, dysexecutive problems in the case of the sentence-to-picture matching task (but also in the sentence-to-word matching task in the case of ambiguous idioms), word comprehension

deficits in the case of the sentence-to-word matching task. Furthermore, RBD patients' performance can be affected by attentional, spatial, or perceptive deficits. When there is a suboptimal processing of critical elements, subjects might be particularly likely to choose the literal interpretation, which is the less demanding one. Other paradigms have been used, such as plausibility judgments or word monitoring, but they are difficult for aphasic patients, unless their deficit is very mild. Therefore, it is reasonable to check idiom performance with different tasks in order to obtain converging evidence.

3. The particular type and structure of an idiom is of some relevance. Patients show a different pattern of performance with ambiguous and unambiguous items, decomposable and non-decomposable idioms, verbal and nominal idiomatic phrases.

In conclusion, idioms are difficult for neurological or psychiatric patients, although the degree of difficulty varies among subjects and differs depending on the type of task and type of idiom. There are at least two contributing factors: aphasic patients find it difficult to perform the linguistic analysis, which depletes their cognitive resources; prefrontal patients fail to inhibit/suppress the literal meaning or to activate the figurative one. The reported data do not support the right hemisphere hypothesis; they also challenge the psycholinguistic hypothesis, which posits that idioms are simply long, morphologically complex words. Finally, they unequivocally show that metaphors and idioms *cannot* be considered together as a single type of figurative language, but that even within the idiom class, it is necessary to distinguish among different expressions.

References

1. Gibbs RW (1999) Figurative language. In: Wilson R, Keil F (eds) The MIT encyclopedia of the cognitive science. MIT Press, Cambridge, MA, pp 314-315
2. Nunberg G, Sag IA, Wasow T (1994) Idioms. Language 70:491-538
3. Cacciari C, Glucksberg S (1995) Understanding idioms: do visual images reflect figurative meanings? Eur J Cogn Psychol 7:283-305
4. Glucksberg S (2001) Understanding figurative language. Oxford University Press, Oxford
5. Gibbs RW, Nayak, NP, Cutting C (1989) How to kick the bucket and not decompose: analyzability and idiom processing. J Mem Lang 28:576-593
6. Gibbs RW, Gonzales GP (1985) Syntactic frozenness in processing and remembering idioms. Cognition 20:243-259
7. Colombo L (1993) The comprehension of ambiguous idioms in context. In: Cacciari C, Tabossi P (eds) Idioms: processing, structure, and interpretation. Lawrence Erlbaum, Hillsdale, pp 163-200
8. Colombo L (1998) Role of context in the comprehension of ambiguous Iitalian idioms. In: Hillert D (ed) Syntax and semantics, vol 31. Academic Press, New York, pp 379-404
9. Giora R, Zaidel E, Soroker N et al (2000) Differential effects of right- and left-hemisphere damage on understanding sarcasm and metaphor. Metaphor & Symbol 15:63-83
10. Nenonen M, Niemi J, Laine M (2002) Representation and processing of idioms: evidence from aphasia. Journal of Neurolinguistics 15:43-58

6

11. Papagno C, Genoni A (2004) The role of syntactic competence in idiom comprehension: a study on aphasic patients. Journal of Neurolinguistics 17:371-382
12. Papagno C, Tabossi P, Colombo M, Zampetti P (2004) Idiom comprehension in aphasic patients. Brain Lang 89:226-234
13. Rinaldi MC, Marangolo P, Baldassarri F (2004) Metaphor comprehension in right brain-damaged patients with visuo-verbal material: a dissociation (re)considered. Cortex 40:479-490
14. Burgess C, Chiarello C (1996) Neurocognitive mechanisms underlying metaphor comprehension and other figurative language. Metaphor Symbolic Activity 11:67-84
15. Winner E, Gardner H (1977) The comprehension of metaphor in brain-damaged patients. Brain 100:717-729
16. Stachowiak F, Huber W, Poeck K, Kerschensteiner M (1977) Text comprehension in aphasia. Brain Lang 4:177-195
17. Van Lancker D, Kempler D (1987) Comprehension of familiar phrases by left but not by right hemisphere damaged patients. Brain Lang 32:265-277
18. Kempler D, Van Lancker D, Marchman V, Bates E (1999) Idiom comprehension in children and adults with unilateral brain damage. Dev Neuropsychol 15:327-349
19. Papagno C, Curti R, Rizzo S et al (2006) Is the right hemisphere involved in idiom comprehension? A neuropsychological study. Neuropsychology 20:598-606
20. Tompkins CA, Boada R, McGarry K (1992) The access and processing of familiar idioms by brain-damaged and normally aging adults. J Speech Hear Res 35:626-637
21. Swinney DA, Cutler A (1979) The access and processing of idiomatic expressions. J Verb Learn Verb Behav 18:523-534
22. Cacciari C, Reati F, Colombo M-R et al (2006) The comprehension of ambiguous idioms in aphasic patients. Neuropsychologia 44:1305-1314
23. Papagno C, Caporali A (2007) Testing idiom comprehension in aphasic patients: the effects of task and idiom type. Brain Lang 100:208-220
24. Hillert D (2004) Spared access to idiomatic and literal meanings: a single-case approach. Brain Lang 89:207-215
25. Oliveri M, Romero L, Papagno C (2004) Left but not right temporal lobe involvement in opaque idiom comprehension: a repetitive transcranial magnetic stimulation study. J Cognit Neurosc 16:848-855
26. Fogliata A, Rizzo S, Reati F et al (2007) The time corse of idiom processing. Neuropsychologia 45:3215-3222
27. Rizzo S, Sandrini M, Papagno C (2007) The dorsolateral prefrontal cortex in idiom interpretation: an rTMS study. Brain Res Bull 71:523-528
28. Papagno C, Vallar G (2001) Understanding metaphor and idioms: a single case neuropsychological study in a subject with Down syndrome. J Intern Neuropsychol Soc 7:516-528
29. Romero Lauro LJ, Tettamanti M, Cappa SF, Papagno C (2008) Idiom comprehension: a prefrontal task? Cerebral Cortex 18:162-170
30. Zempleni MZ, Haverkort M, Renken R, Sotwe LA (2007) Evidence for bilateral involvement in idiom comprehension: an fMRI study. NeuroImage 34:1280-1291
31. Hillert DG, Buracas GT (2009) The neural substrates of spoken idiom comprehension. Lang Cognit Proc 24:1370-1391
32. Huber-Okrainec J, Blaser SE, Dennis M (2005) Idiom comprehension deficits in relation to corpus calosum agenesis and hypoplasia in children with spina bifida meningomyelocele. Brain Lang 93:349-368.
33. Kempler D, Van Lancker D, Read S (1988) Proverb and idiom comprehension in Alzheimer disease. Alzheimer Dis Assoc Dis 2:38-49
34. Papagno C (2001) Comprehension of metaphors and idioms in patients with Alzheimer's disease: a longitudinal study. Brain 124:1450-1460

35. Papagno C, Cappa SF, Garavaglia P et al (1995) La comprensione non letterale del linguaggio: taratura su soggetti normali. Archivio di Psicologia, Neurologia e Psichiatria 56:402-420
36. Papagno C, Lucchelli F, Muggia S, Rizzo S (2003) Idiom comprehension in Alzheimer's disease: the role of the central executive. Brain 126:2419-2430
37. Rassiga C, Lucchelli F, Crippa F, Papagno C (2009) Ambiguous idiom comprehension in Alzheimer's disease. J Clin Exp Neuropsychol 31:402-411
38. Titone D, Holzman PS, Levy DL (2002) Idiom processing in schizophrenia: literal implausibility saves the day for idiom priming. J Abnorm Psychol 111:313-320
39. Iakimova G, Passerieux C, Hardy-Baylé M-C (2006) Interpretation of ambiguous idiomatic statements in schizophrenic and depressive patients. Evidence for common and differential cognitive patterns. Psychopathology 39:277-285
40. Tavano A, Sponda S, Fabbro F et al (2008) Specific linguistic and pragmatic deficits in Italian patients with schizophrenia. Schiz Res 102:53-62
41. Schettino A, Romero Lauro LJ, Crippa F et al (2010) The comprehension of idiomatic expressions in schizophrenic patients. Neuropsychologia 48:1032-1040

Anticipatory Mechanisms in Idiom Comprehension: Psycholinguistic and Electrophysiological Evidence

7

P. Canal, F. Vespignani, N. Molinaro, C. Cacciari

7.1 Introduction

Idiomatic expressions are highly pervasive in everyday language: as Jackendoff [1] pointed out, in American English there are as many words as there are *multi-word expressions* (i.e., word strings listed in semantic memory, as proverbs, clichés, idioms, phrasal verbs, etc.), roughly around 80 000 [2]. If, indeed, *multi-word* expressions are so pervasive in everyday language, no theory of language can ignore them. In fact, during the last few decades a consistent body of research on the comprehension and production of idioms has accumulated in psycholinguistics [3-5] and, more recently, in the cognitive neurosciences (e.g., [6], Mado Proverbio, this volume).

In this chapter, we examine the role of anticipatory[1] mechanisms in the comprehension of idiomatic expressions. These multi-word strings are characterized by the fact that their meaning is conventionalized and their constituents are bound together with a pre-defined order.

[1] For sake of brevity we consider the concepts of prediction, anticipation, or forward-looking as interchangeable: actually they are not, but the distinction between them is beyond the scope of this chapter.

C. Cacciari (✉)
Department of Biomedical Sciences, University of Modena and Reggio Emilia, Modena, Italy

7.2 What an Idiomatic Expression Is (and Is Not)

An idiom is a string of constituents whose meaning is not necessarily derived from that of the constituent parts. Idiomatic expressions are stored in semantic memory together with a variety of knowledge that includes not only word meanings and concepts but also word strings that people learn: movies, book titles, song titles, lyrics, lines of poetry, clichés, idioms, proverbs, and so forth [7]. Idioms belong to the realm of *conventionalized* expressions that speakers use within a linguistic community, and probably they represent the largest part of it: as the language philosopher John Searle [8] put it, in everyday conversation people seem to adhere to the following adagio: *Speak idiomatically unless there is some special reason not to* (p. 50).

For a long time, idioms were seen as totally arbitrary associations between form and meaning. This assumption has been an obstacle to understanding the variegated nature of idiomatic expressions [9]. Idiom heterogeneity can be exemplified as follows: some idiomatic expressions convey semantically plausible actions (e.g., *kick the bucket*, *spill the beans*), just as others represent implausible actions (*wear one's heart on one's sleeve*, *to be in seventh heaven*); some idioms have unusual if not ungrammatical forms (*by and large*, *trip the light fantastic*), whereas others are syntactically well-formed (*break the ice*, *pull strings*); some idioms are semantically ambiguous and can be interpreted literally as well as figuratively[2] (*a red eye*, *hold the aces*), whereas others have only a figurative interpretation (*a wolf in sheep's clothing*, *have a chance in hell*); some of them are syntactically flexible and allow syntactic transformations (e.g., passivization, such as in *the strings were pulled by his parents in order to get that job*; nominalization, such as in *his laying down of the law so harshly hurt Joanna*; insertion, such as in *he left no legal stone unturned looking for the guilty*), whereas others behave like frozen blocks that lose their figurative meaning if changed. Also the semantic contribution of the idiom's constituents[3] to the idiomatic meaning differs: some idioms are semantically opaque[4] (*kick the bucket*, *chew the fat*) while others are more semantically transparent (*skate on thin ice*). However, since we know the meaning of an idiom we can overestimate how much the idiomatic meaning is semantically transparent. In other words, we may illusorily assume that there is a systematic mapping between literal and figurative meanings [11].

---

[2] Nonetheless in these ambiguous expressions there is almost always a dominant meaning that usually is the idiomatic meaning.

[3] The assumption of Wasow et al. [9], which led Gibbs and colleagues to develop the decomposition hypothesis [10], is that *pieces of idioms typically have identifiable meanings that combine to produce the meaning as a whole. Of course these meanings are not the literal meanings of the parts. Rather, idiomatic meanings are generally derived from literal meanings in conventionalized, but not entirely arbitrary ways* (p.109). The idea of regarding idioms as compositional strings did not find clear empirical evidence in psycholinguistics. The only positive results come from studies on post-perceptive interpretive processes (e.g., semantic acceptability judgments, paraphrase production or judgments).

[4] A semantically transparent idiom is one in which the meaning of the expression can be derived from the literal meanings of the constituents or from the rhetoric structure of the idiom.

The metaphoric origin of some idioms can be still perceivable (e.g., *pull the string*, *carry coals to Newcastle*; for a discussion on quasi-metaphorical idioms see [12, 13]) and it may have some consequences for linguistic processing, if we consider interpretive tasks [14]. But the evidence on an on-line impact of idioms' semantic transparency on the time required to recognize and activate the idiom meanings is still scarce and inconclusive. This does not mean that the semantic properties of the idiom's constituent words are irrelevant also for idiomatic expressions that are completely opaque. As Wasow, Sag, and Nunberg [7, 9, 15, 16] pointed out, the reason why we cannot say *He lay kicking the bucket all week* resides in the type of action that the verb *kick* denotes, which is a discrete action. Similarly, we can say *He didn't spill a single bean*, because *beans* are numerable entities.

It is worth noting also the differences between idioms, metaphors, and proverbs. Idiomatic expressions differ from *metaphors*, even though some idioms diachronically derive from them, since metaphors (also the more conventionalized ones) do not have a unique standardized meaning in the linguistic community, but can convey more than one meaning. Idioms, instead, do have a unique meaning that can be specialized by context but not changed. Then, idioms differ from proverbs since the latter are full sentences, temporarily undefined, signaled by specific grammatical, phonetic, and/or rhetorical patterns, or by a binary structure. Proverbs are used as general comments to shared communicative situations, and are generally true statements, both literally and figuratively[5].

7.3 Semantic Forward-looking Mechanisms in Idiom Comprehension

The identity of many idiomatic expressions can be determined in advance, or predicted with reasonable confidence, on the basis of a certain amount of input that varies depending on how many words have to be read or perceived before they call to mind the corresponding idiom. For instance, if we ask participants to complete sentence fragments of increasing length as, for instance, *John was ...*, we collect the most different kinds of completions (e.g., *walking*, *cool*, *American*, *sad* etc.). If we add a constituent (*breathing*), and we ask for the completion of *John was breathing...* people will complete it with a smaller number of alternatives, e.g. *deeply*, *hard*, etc. When we ask for the completion *John was breathing down ...* a large proportion of people will do so with *his neck*, and almost all participants will complete the sentence with *neck* if presented with *John was breathing down his....* According to the terminology proposed by Cacciari and Tabossi [19], this type of idiom is *predictable* in that it is recognized as an idiom before the last constituent. In contrast, there are idioms that are *unpredictable* insofar as their idiomatic meaning is recognized only after the last constituent of the idiom string has been processed (as for instance in *John broke the ice*).

[5] An elaboration on the differences between collocations and idioms can be found in [17] and [18].

The recognition of the idiomatic nature of an idiom string is crucial for one of the hypotheses on idioms comprehension, the configuration hypothesis (CH)[6]. This hypothesis was originally proposed by Cacciari and Tabossi [19] and assumes that the literal meaning of the constituent words of the expressions are activated at least until the sequence of words is recognized as an idiomatic configuration. In a sentence containing a predictable idiom, such as *Jessie took the bull by the horns*, the constituent that triggers idiom recognition is defined as the *recognition point* of the idiom (operationally, it is the constituent that causes a dramatic increase in the probability of the idiomatic completion *bull*). The recognition point differs for different idioms and it might also vary for the same idiom depending on the sentential context in which the idiom is embedded. Idioms are particularly sensitive to the preceding contextual information, and even a minimal context might anticipate the recognition of an idiom. As Peterson et al. [21] noted, two-noun phrases such as *The soccer player* and *the old man* elicit radically different semantic representations when inserted before the verb phrase *kicked the bucket*.

According to the CH, the same lexical units that are involved during literal sentences comprehension are also involved in the comprehension of idioms. In other words, only one type of processing (literal processing) operates in idiom comprehension until, after the recognition point of the idiomatic expression, the meaning of the configuration is retrieved from semantic memory: literal processing and whole-phrase meaning retrieval coexist in idiom comprehension. This process may require some time to be brought to an end, especially with strings that are non-predictable before the end, or for idioms embedded in neutral contexts [19]. The CH has found supporting evidence in several studies on comprehension [21-26]. Recent studies on idiom production found evidence compatible with the general claims of the CH [27-29]: for instance, Cutting and Bock [27] using a speech error induction technique, found that participants produced a relevant number of *idiom blends* that revealed joint syntactic-semantic effects often originating from the similarity between literal and idiomatic meanings (e.g., *Swallow the bullet* instead of *Bite the bullet*; *The road to Chicago is straight as a pancake*, an expression that blends *straight as an arrow* and *flat as a pancake*). These results suggest that idioms are not produced as phrasal units with semantically empty constituents [20, 30], but are semantically analyzed and syntactically processed [10, 21, 28].

The recognition point of an idiomatic expression is usually operationalized on the basis of off-line completion tests through which a *cloze probability* value [31-33] is assigned. A well-established result in psycholinguistic literature is that, in neutral contexts, the meaning of predictable idioms (the ones that can be completed idiomatically

---

[6] This hypothesis was conceived as a reply to the classical lexical representation hypothesis [20] which assumed that idioms are represented as long words, *multi-word lexical entries*, listed in the lexicon, together with all the other words; their meaning would be retrieved in the same way as any other single word. Authors proposed that the processing of the two meanings, both literal and figurative, starts simultaneously as soon as the first word of the expression is perceived. However, the process of recognizing the idiom is faster than the computation of the corresponding literal string, because it depends on the retrieval of the global meaning of the expression as a long word, bringing the literal analysis to an end.

before the last constituent) is already activated at the end of the string. On the other hand, the results are far from homogeneous with unpredictable idioms: methodological differences, specific to the categorization of predictable *vs* unpredictable idioms, can partially explain this non-homogeneity (for other concurring factors, see [14, 23]).

What is the difference, if any, between anticipating the literal continuation or the idiomatic continuation of a sentence? On the one hand, it seems intuitive that the frequency of co-occurrence of the constituents that form a familiar idiomatic string is higher than that of words that freely occur in literal language. Therefore, since the idiomatic constituents are *bound* together, it is reasonable to suppose that semantic forward-looking mechanisms might be different in literal *vs* non-literal language. For instance, consider *Jen took the bull ... vs Jen spread her toast with...* In the first case, the fragment may call to mind the idiom *take the bull by the horns* and its corresponding meaning. In this example, only one idiom matches the fragment, even if we cannot exclude less frequent literal completions (*Jen took the bull to the veterinary*). In the literal sentence there is more than one constituent that may match the verb argument of *spread* even if some constituents have higher cloze probabilities than others (e.g., *butter vs jam*).

Altmann and Kamide [34] and other scholars [35, 36] showed that literal constraints might be very strong and might affect linguistic processing in early stages. While listening to sentences such as *The boy will move the cake* or *The boy will eat the cake*, we are presented with a visual scene with only one eatable thing (a cake). The eye movements recorded 50 ms after the onset of the verb significantly differ according to the sentence content. With the verb *move*, the first saccade on the picture of a cake starts 127 ms *after* the onset of *cake*, and with the verb *eat* the first saccade takes place 85 ms *before* the *cake* onset. In other words, the information derived from the verb guides the eye movements toward any object that satisfies the selectional restrictions of the verb [34]. Trueswell et al. [36] proposed that sentence processing is highly predictive: *any and all available information is recruited to the task of predicting subsequent input* (p. 262). This mechanism activates the verb's argument representations and evaluates those arguments not only against the current linguistic input but against the anticipated context as well.

However, literal and figurative expressions differ in an important aspect, the compositionality of meaning. In other words, even if we have a literal and an idiomatic sentence whose post-verbal constituents have a similarly high cloze probability, the mechanisms underlying the comprehension of the two sentences still might differ. In the comprehension of sentences with an idiom the meanings of the idiomatic constituents are incrementally activated and together contribute to build the meaning representation of the sentence only until the idiom is recognized. After this point, the idiomatic meaning[7] is retrieved from semantic memory and is integrated in the sentence representation. For literal sentences, a compositional strategy should suffice to construct the sentential meaning.

---

[7] Results from Peterson et al. [21] suggest that the syntactic analysis of the string is carried on, even after the recognition of the idiomatic nature of the string. This would be compatible with evidence showing that the literal meaning of the constituent words might be activated even when the idiomatic meaning is already retrieved [19].

7

The seminal work of Kutas and Hillyard [37, for overviews, see: 38-40] in the early 1980s showed that the human brain is very sensitive to the distributional properties of language. The N400, discovered by Kutas and Hillyard [37, 41][8], is a negative component of scalp-recorded event-related potentials (ERP) peaking around 400 ms from stimulus presentation and characterized by a central-posterior, slightly right lateralized, scalp distribution. The amplitude of the N400[9] is sensitive to how much the preceding context constrains the predictability or ease of integration of an upcoming word [44, 45].

As Kutas and Federmeier [39] noted, the brain uses contextual information *to predict* (i.e., *anticipate and prepare for*) *the perceptual and semantic features of items likely to appear, in order to comprehend the intended meaning of a sentence at the fast speed with which it usually comes* (p. 466). This strategy meets a more general principle of cognitive economy: the language comprehension system makes use of all the information it can *as early as it can to constrain the search through semantic memory and facilitate the processing of the item(s) more likely to appear. Such a predictive strategy allows for more efficient processing when the expectation is upheld* (p. 467).

As we said, idiomatic expressions are well-suited for investigating the role of semantic forward-looking mechanisms. However, despite the thousands of ERP studies on the comprehension of words and sentences in their many different aspects (phonology, orthography, syntax, semantics), ERP studies on idiomatic expressions are very few, essentially six[10] [46-51].

The first ERP studies, conducted by Strandburg et al. [46, 47], showed the relevance of context on idiom processing. These authors measured the ERPs time-locked to the second word of visually presented word pairs that could be literal (e.g., *vicious dog*), idiomatic (e.g., *vicious circle*), or non-sensical (e.g., *square wind*). Healthy and patient participants were asked to perform a semantic acceptability task. In order to correctly identify the meaning of the word pairs, one has to retrieve the figurative meaning of the figurative pair from semantic memory. As we know from the literature, autistic patients tend to interpret idioms literally and schizophrenics are deficient in using contextual information. In fact, Strandburg and colleagues found different N400 effects in healthy *vs* the patient participants: healthy participants showed an increase of the N400 amplitude from the idiomatic to the literal to the nonsense condition. The second word of the idiomatic pair elicited a reduced negativity compared to the literal condition. The two patient groups differed: schizophrenic patients showed an increased negativity for the N400 on the second word whereas autistic patients did not

---

8 In the seminal study by Kutas and Hillyard, participants were visually presented with sentences that ended with a semantically congruous last constituent (*I take my coffee with cream and SUGAR*) or with a semantically incongruous word (*I take my coffee with cream and DOG*). The observed negativity in the EEG signal was larger for the incongruous ending (*DOG*) than for the congruous one (*SUGAR*). For overviews on language-related ERPs see [42, 43].

9 The N400 is not the only language-related component: there is a large number of studies that have investigated the different components associated with language processing [42, 43].

10 In general there are few ERP studies on figurative language.

show any negativity at all. A critical factor of these studies, acknowledged by the authors, concerns the P300 component, a well-studied ERP component that partially overlaps with the N400 in a similar time window. In both studies, some differences in the amplitude of the P300 in the different groups emerged. In autistic patients, the P300 component was larger than in healthy participants, whereas schizophrenic patients showed a reduced positivity with respect to the control group. However, it might be argued that the N400 differences are the product of an interaction between these two overlapping components, with the N400 increasing as the P300 is reduced. The authors employed principal component analysis (PCA) to address this issue and showed two different components, identified as N400 (in the 320- to 580-ms time-window) and P300 (in the 450- to 850-ms time-window). The P300s are a large family of functionally distinct components and the PCA conducted by Strandburg and colleagues cannot argue against the possibility that an earlier positive component overlapping the N400 affects the amplitude of the observed negativities.

Moreno et al. [48] tested English-Spanish bilinguals. They were asked to read literal or figurative English sentences ending with: (a) expected high cloze probability words (i.e., literal completions or proverb/idiom completions); (b) within-language lexical switches (i.e., English synonyms of the expected completions); (c) code switches (i.e., translations into Spanish of the expected completions). Within-language lexical switches elicited a large N400 in literal and figurative contexts and a late positivity in the figurative context. In contrast, code switches elicited a positivity that began at about 450 ms post-word-onset and continued into the 650- to 850-ms time window. In summary, the amplitude of the N400 was affected by the predictability of the lexical item regardless of prior context, and the latency of the N400 to lexical switches was affected by English vocabulary proficiency.

In Zhou et al.'s study [49] idioms were visually presented to healthy participants. Chinese four-character idioms have a fixed structure in which neither characters nor their order can be modified, while the experimental manipulation consisted in the replacement of the fourth character, triggering both a semantic and a syntactic violation. The participants were asked to judge whether the last constituent was appropriate. The ERPs showed that reading the wrong character had different effects in different time windows: a right frontal and right parietal negativity between 125 and 150 ms; a centrally distributed negativity between 300 and 400 ms; and a positive deflection in the left occipital-temporal-parietal scalp sites. The first effect (ERHN, *early right hemispheric negativity*) might be part of an initial stage of syntactic processing since there was a violation of word category; the second, on the N400 component, could represent the integration of syntactic and semantic analysis of the stimulus; the third, on the P600 component, might reflect a re-analysis process that tries to integrate the critical word in the context. Unfortunately, this study lacked a literal control condition. Anyway, a visual inspection of the unsubtracted waveforms might suggest the presence of a positive peak between 320 and 380 ms for the idiomatic condition rather than a negative deflection for the incongruous word.

In the French study conducted by Laurent et al. [50] the authors used familiar idiomatic expressions with both a literal and figurative interpretation (e.g., *rendre les armes*) out of context: first, the onset of the expression was presented on the screen (*rendre les*), and then it was followed by the remainder of the expression (*armes*). A word semantically related or unrelated to the idiom's meaning was presented 300 ms later and participants were asked to decide whether or not the target was semantically related to the meaning of the utterance. The ERPs were time-locked to the last word of the idiom and included the target presentation. The main experimental manipulation was the degree of saliency of the idioms employed: *strongly salient* idioms were compared with *weakly salient* idioms. The notion of salience comes from the pragmatic tradition and has been recently adapted to the context of figurative language by Giora (for an overview, see [52, 53]). This notion is somewhat puzzling since it is rather vague and partially overlaps with the notion of familiarity, of meaning dominance, and syntactic/semantic *well-formedness*. In Laurent et al.'s study, it is not clear what was meant by a strongly salient or weakly salient idiom: it seems reasonable to assume that the authors intended a figurative dominant meaning. It should, in any case, be noted that the effect of the predictability of the last constituent was not controlled for, which might be a serious confound. In fact, the predictability of the last constituent was 45.5% for weakly salient idioms and 58.8% for strongly salient idioms. Since, according to the authors, the processing of salient idioms should not differ from the processing of literal language, strongly salient idiomatic strings and literal expressions should show similar ERP waveforms (however, since the idioms were ambiguous and presented out of context, we cannot know whether participants activated both meanings or only the dominant meaning). In any case, strongly and weakly salient idioms should differ. However, Laurent et al. only showed a difference in the amplitude of the N400 of weakly *vs* strongly salient idioms. Moreover, the reported P600 had a morphology different from the one typically described in the literature.

These few studies on the electrophysiological correlates of idiom comprehension had important limitations. For instance, the ERPs were always recorded at the offset of the idiomatic string, which in some studies coincided also with the last word of the trial's presentation, in which ERPs modulations in the N400 time window were reported. In fact, an N400-like component, *wrap-up negativity*, is usually observed for the last word of a sentence. It is considered to reflect a final re-processing of the structure and meaning of the sentence.

7.4 An ERP Study on the Comprehension of Idiomatic Expressions in Italian: The N400 and the Electrophysiological Correlate of Categorical Expectations

The aim of our study [51] was to assess the ERP correlates of the comprehension of highly predictable word strings. In the theoretical framework of the CH, we assumed that recognition of the idiomatic nature of the expression was a prerequisite for accessing the idiomatic meaning. This should surface in different waveforms before *vs* after the recognition of the idiomatic nature of the string. We identified a set of familiar unambiguous idioms ($n = 87$) predictable before the offset of the expression.

The *recognition point* (RP) was determined as the word after which the string was continued idiomatically in at least 65% of the cases. The mean cloze probability value was 86% (range 65–100%). Each idiomatic expression was inserted in a neutral context that ended with non-idiomatic constituents to avoid any *wrap-up* effect on the idiom. Three conditions were designed:

1. In the *idiomatic* condition, the idiomatic expression was presented in its canonical form (*Giorgio aveva un buco allo stomaco quella mattina; Giorgio had a hole in his stomach that morning*, i.e., was hungry).
2. In the *substitution* condition, the recognition point of the idiom was substituted with an idiom-unrelated word (of the same grammatical category) that fitted in the preceding context (*Giorgio aveva un dolore allo stomaco quella mattina; Giorgio had a pain in his stomach that morning*).
3. In the *expectancy-violation condition*, the constituent after the recognition point was substituted (*Giorgio aveva un buco sulla camica quella mattina; Giorgio had a hole in his shirt that morning*) with a word of the same grammatical category that again fitted in the preceding context. All the sentences were syntactically and semantically well-formed. The sentences (29 per condition) were displayed word by word at the center of the screen (for 300 ms with an inter-stimulus interval of 300 ms). The participants ($n = 50$) were required to read for comprehension (comprehension questions on fillers were inserted every 10 sentences on average)[11].

A consistent bulk of evidence coming from studies on literal processing demonstrated that the linguistic system is sensitive to the co-occurrence of words; therefore, the ERPs might be sensitive to word co-occurrences even before the activation of the idiomatic meaning: in particular at the recognition point (the point after which the idiomatic nature of the string is recognized) of long idioms such as those used in the study. At the subsequent word (RP+1), the waveforms might show a qualitatively different pattern, since the linguistic input has been recognized as an idiom at this point.

The waveforms at the recognition point of the idiom had a scalp distribution and timing compatible with an N400 that can be explained in cloze probability terms. The results of off-line completion questionnaires support the idea that participants were sensitive to the co-occurrence of the upcoming words: the proportion of idiomatic completions at RP (0.37) was smaller than the proportion at RP+1 (0.86) but still remarkable. In any case, participants might have developed a sense of familiarity for the words presented until that point even before full recognition of the idiom, and this was indexed by an N400 for the substitution condition. After the recognition point, a change in the morphology of the waveforms occurred characterized by a more posterior topographic distribution, with the effect being present on more distal sites (PO3-PO4) and not only on the typical N400 sites. In the waveform elicited by the idiomat-

---

[11] The EEG signal was amplified and digitized continuously with a 30 active electrodes system (BioSemi) placed on the scalp according to a 10-20 standard system. Epochs containing the two target words were extracted with a duration of 1500 ms, starting 200 ms prior to the onset of the recognition point (the extracted average waveforms for each participant after artifacts rejection (13.5%) and baseline correction have been subsequently averaged together).

ic condition, there was a positive peak around 300 ms, identified as a P300. In order to assess the exact timing of the effects at RP and at RP+1, we conducted several analyses (see [51]). In one of them, we examined the values of the *t*-tests conducted on the average voltage of a centroparietal cluster of sites (C3, Cz, C4, CP1, CP2, P3, Pz, P4) on every subsequent 10-ms time windows from the presentation of the two target words. This analysis showed that the two conditions significantly diverged after 320 ms from the RP presentation; at RP+1 the difference between idiomatic and violation conditions was significant at around 260 ms.

The latency analysis, together with the observed morphological differences of the unsubtracted waveforms, converged to support the claim that the observed waveforms did not derive from a modulation of the same component (N400). Indeed, the N400 has a quite stable spatial distribution and time development. The N400 slightly changes its timing and spatial development when different groups of participants or different kinds of stimuli presentations (auditory *vs* visually presented, sentences *vs* words *vs* pictures) are compared. Linguistic material manipulation (lexical word frequency, word position in the sentence, cloze probability, etc.) typically affects the amplitude of the N400, and not the spatial-temporal characteristics (for related claims, see reviews in [39, 40]).

Evidence consistent with our interpretation of a P300 at RP+1 comes from an ERP study on antonymous word pairs (e.g., *black-white*, *hot-cold*); experiment 1 in [54]). Previous studies [54, 55] showed that if we compare *The opposite of white is black* with a sentence ending with a wrong antonym (*yellow* or *nice*), *nice* elicits an N400 that is larger than the N400 for *yellow* since *nice* is not a color and thus it does not share the same semantic category of the most expected word. In contrast, Roehm et al. [54] showed a P300 for the right element of the antonymous word pair that might overlap with the N400 but showed a scalp distribution and morphology which differed from what is typical of the N400. In a second experiment of the same study, an N400 emerged but with a different paradigm, namely, with a lexical decision task on the second word. No P300 was found probably because the meta-linguistic task minimized the need for comprehension-related predictive mechanisms.

As we said, the results that emerged from our study at RP+1 were very similar to those of Roehm et al. (experiment 1, [54]). This similarity indirectly supports our interpretation of the results as a P300 effect elicited by processing the idiomatic constituents after (and only after) the recognition of the idiomatic nature of the string.

In summary, our study showed the presence of two different cognitive markers associated with two different stages of idiom comprehension:

- at the recognition point (RP), a centrally distributed N400 elicited by the substitution condition, congruent with the N400 literature on literal sentence processing, stands for the development of some "sense of familiarity" of the idiom before the recognition point;
- at the word following the recognition point (RP+1), the waveforms diverge earlier (70 ms before). The waveforms associated with the idiomatic condition showed a P300 indexing a different mechanism that comes into play when the idiomatic meaning has been already retrieved.

How can we interpret our P300[12]? Kok [60] proposed a functional interpretation of the P300 that perfectly captures our results. According to Kok, there is a general consensus that the P300 is evoked after the stimulus has been evaluated even on the basis of partial information. The P300 amplitude might reflect the *attentional capacity invested in categorizing of task relevant [...] events. Event categorization is [...] a process that leads to the decision that the external stimulus matches (or does not match) with an internal representation of a specific event or category of stimuli* ([60], p. 571). This conceptualization of the P300 has something in common with the idea of interpreting it as the signature of a template-matching process [61]: when participants are asked to detect a stimulus, they develop a representation of the target or template of the stimulus. The P300 amplitude is larger when the incoming information is closer to that template. This hypothesis has some support also in language studies which demonstrated that the P300s are sensitive to the relative familiarity of words [62]. Kok concluded that the *P300 reflects processes that underlie recognition processes (i.e. the awareness that a stimulus belongs or does not belong to the category of a certain memorized target event)* (p. 573). Why should this framework be relevant for interpreting our P300 effect? Our hypothesis is that the P300 indexes the process that starts soon after the recognition of the idiom and after its meaning retrieval: the reader might look for a match between the idiomatic expression represented in its canonical form in semantic memory (the *template*) and the upcoming constituents. In our study, as in the antonym study, a P300 is evoked by the attended word. What these types of expression share is that the expectancy for the last constituents is categorical and not probabilistic. The categorical nature of the expectations derives from the semantic memory representation of these word strings. The P300 obtained during idiomatic processing might reflect the monitoring of the match between the activated configuration and the constituents that occurred after the recognition point.

What are the implications of these results for idiom comprehension theories? The most important is that the processing of idiomatic constituents, before and after recognition of the expressions, differs and has different electrophysiological correlates, which indirectly supports the CH [19]. More generally, this study highlights the presence of different anticipation mechanisms that might come into play not only in idiom processing but also in all the expressions that have a *bound* representation (collocations, clichés, song or book titles, etc.).

[12] The P300s form a family of positive components that usually are not related to linguistic processing. The P300 is one of the most studied ERP components in the ERP literature, and it has been shown to be sensitive to different cognitive aspects of stimulus processing. The definition of the functional role of the P300s is far from trivial because different P300s have been found to have different functional roles. It is impossible to summarize the P300 literature (see [56-60]).

7

7.5 Conclusions

In this chapter, we argued that idioms, a linguistic phenomenon that has been underestimated, provide an interesting case for testing predictive linguistic processing. This is due to the fact that their identity can be predicted before the end of the expression based on an amount of input that varies depending on how much of the string is necessary before it is possible to retrieve their meaning from semantic memory. In other words, the processes involved in idiom comprehension exemplify the functioning of our *proactive brain* [63].

References

1. Jackendoff R (1995) The boundaries of the lexicon. In: Everaert M, van den Linden E, Schenk E, Schreuder E (eds) Idioms: structural and psychological perspectives. Erlbaum, Hillsdale, NJ, pp 133-166
2. Pollio H, Barlow J, Fine H, Pollio M (1977) Metaphor and the poetics of growth: figurative language in psychology, psychotherapy and education. Erlbaum, Hillsdale, NJ
3. Cacciari C, Tabossi P (eds) (1993) Idioms. Processing, structure and interpretation. Erlbaum, Hillsdale, NJ
4. Everaert M, van der Linden EJ, Schenk A, Schreuder R (eds) (1995) Idioms: structural and Psychological Perspectives. Erlbaum, Hillsdale, NJ
5. Bobrow S, Bell S (1973) On catching on to idiomatic expressions. Mem Cogn 1: 343-346
6. Katz AN (2006) (ed) Special issue: metaphor and the brain. Metaphor and Symbol 21:4
7. Nunberg G, Sag I A, Wasow T (1994) Idioms. Language 70:491-538
8. Searle JR (1979) Expression and meaning: studies in the theory of speech acts. Cambridge University Press, Cambridge
9. Wasow T, Sag I, Nunberg G (1983) Idioms: an interim report. In: Hattori S, Inoue K (eds) Proceedings of the XIIIth International Congress of Linguistics, Tokyo, 1983, pp 102-105
10. Gibbs RW, Nayak NP, Cutting C (1989) How to kick the bucket and not decompose: analyzability and idiom processing. J Mem Lang 22:577-590
11. Keysar B, Bly B (1995) Intuitions of the transparency of idioms: can one keep a secret by spilling the beans? J Mem Lang 1:89-109
12. Cacciari C, Glucksberg S (1991) Understanding idiomatic expressions. The contribution of word meanings. In: Simpson G (ed) Understanding word and sentence. Elsevier, Amsterdam, pp 217-240
13. Cacciari C (1993) The place of idioms in a literal and metaphorical world. In: Cacciari C, Tabossi P (eds) Idioms. Processing, structure and Interpretation. Erlbaum, Hillsdale, NJ, pp 27-55
14. Libben MR, Titone DA (2008) The multidetermined nature of idiom processing. Mem Cogn 36:1103-1121
15. Glucksberg S (1993) Idiom meaning and allusional content. In: Cacciari C, Tabossi P (eds) Idioms: processing, structure, and interpretation. Erlbaum, Hillsdale, NJ, pp 3-26
16. Hamblin J L, Gibbs R W (1999) Why you can't kick the bucket as you slowly die. Verbs in idiom comprehension. J Psycholinguist Res 28:25-39
17. Nenonen M, Niemi S (2007) (eds) Collocation and idioms 1. Hoensuu Univeristy Press, Hoensuu

18. Fellbaum C (2007) (ed) Idioms and collocations. From corpus to electronic lexical resource. Continuum, Birmingham
19. Cacciari C, Tabossi P (1988) The comprehension of idioms. J Mem Lang 27:668-683
20. Swinney D, Cutler A (1979) The access and processing of idiomatic expressions. J Verbal Learn Verbal Behav 18:523-534
21. Peterson RR, Burgess C, Dell GS, Eberhard KL (2001) Dissociation between syntactic and semantic processing during idiom comprehension. J Exp Psychol Learn Mem Cogn 90:227-234
22. Cacciari C, Padovani R, Corradini P (2007) Exploring the relationship between individuals' speed of processing and their comprehension of spoken idioms. Eur J Cogn Psychol 27:668-683
23. Fanari R, Cacciari C, Tabossi P (2010) Spoken idiom recognition: the role of length and context. Eur J Cogn Psychol (in press)
24. Tabossi P, Zardon F (1993) The activation of idiomatic meaning in spoken language. In: Cacciari C, Tabossi P (eds) Idioms. Processing, structure and interpretation. Erlbaum, Hillsdale, NJ, pp 145-162
25. Tabossi P, Fanari R, Wolf K (2005) Spoken idiom recognition: meaning retrieval and word expectancy. J Psycholinguist Res 34:465-495
26. Titone DA, Connine CN (1994) Comprehension of idiomatic expressions: effect of predictability and literality. J Exp Psychol Learn Mem Cogn 20:1126-1138
27. Cutting JC, Bock K (1997) That's the way the cookie bounces: syntactic and semantic components of experimentally elicited idiom blends. Mem Cogn 25:57-71
28. Sprenger SA, Levelt WJ, Kempen G (2006) Lexical access during the production of idiomatic phrases. J Mem Lang 54:161-184
29. Konopka AE, Bock K (2009) Lexical or syntactic control of sentence formulation? Structural generalization from idiom production. Cogn Psychol 58:68-101
30. Cruse DA (1986) Lexical semantics. Cambridge University Press, New York
31. Bloom PA, Fischler I (1980) Completions norms for 329 sentence contexts. Mem Cogn 8:631-642
32. Miller GA, Selfridge J (1950) Verbal context and the recall of meaningful material. Am J Psychol 63:176-185
33. Taylor WL (1953) "Cloze procedure": a new tool for measuring readability. Journal Q 30:415-433
34. Altmann GTM, Kamide Y (1999) Incremental interpretation of verbs: restricting the domain of subsequent reference. Cognition 73:247-264
35. Eberhard K, Spivey-Knowlton S, Sevivy J, Tanenhaus M (1995) Eye movements as a window into real-time spoken language processing in natural contexts. J Psycholinguist Res 24:409-436
36. Trueswell JC, Tanenhaus MK, Garnsey S (1994) Semantic influences on parsing: Use of thematic role information in syntactic ambiguity resolution. J Mem Lang 33:285-318
37. Kutas M, Hillyard SA (1984) Brain potentials during reading reflect word expectancy and semantic association. Nature 307:161-163
38. Kutas M, Van Petten C (1994) Psycholinguistic evidence electrified: event-related brain potentials investigation. In: Gernsbacher MA (ed) Handbook of psycholinguistics. Academic, New York, pp 83-144
39. Kutas M, Federmeier KD (2000) Electrophysiology reveals semantic memory use in language comprehension. Trends Cogn Sci 4:463-470
40. Kutas M, Van Petten C, Traxler M (2007) Psycholinguistics electrified II (1994-2006). In: Gernsbacher MA, Traxler M (eds) Handbook of psycholinguistics. 2nd edn. Elsevier, New York
41. Kutas M, Hillyard SA (1980) Event-related potentials to semantically inappropriate and surprisingly large words. Biol Psychol 11:99-116

42. Carreiras M, Clifton C (eds) (2005) The on-line study of sentence comprehension. Psychology Press, New York
43. De Vincenzi M, Di Matteo R (2004) Come il cervello comprende il linguaggio. Laterza, Bari
44. De Long KA, Urbach TP, Kutas M (2005) Probabilistic word pre-activation during language comprehension inferred from electrical brain activity. Nat Neurosci 81117-1121
45. Van Berkum JJA, Brown CM, Zwitserlood P et al (2005) Anticipating upcoming words in discourse: evidence from ERPs and Reading Times. J Exp Psychol Learn Mem Cogn 31:443-467
46. Strandburg RJ, Marsh JT, Brown WS et al (1993) Event-related potentials in high-functioning adult autistics: linguistic and nonlinguistic visual information processing tasks. Neuropsychologia 31:413-34
47. Strandburg RJ, Marsh JT, Brown WS et al (1997) Event-related potential correlates of linguistic information processing in schizophrenics. Biol Psychiatry 42:596-608
48. Moreno EM, Federmeier KD, Kutas M (2002) Switching languages, switching palabras (words): an electrophysiological study of code switching. Brain Lang 80:188-207
49. Zhou S, Zhou W, Chen X (2004) Spatiotemporal analysis of ERP during Chinese idiom comprehension. Brain Topogr 17:27-37
50. Laurent JP, Denhières G, Passerieux C et al (2006) On understanding idiomatic language: the salience hypothesis assessed by ERPs. Brain Res 1068:151-60
51. Vespignani F, Canal P, Molinaro N et al (in press) Predictive mechanisms in idiom comprehension. J Cogn Neurosci
52. Giora R (2003) On our minds. Salience, context and figurative language. Oxford University Press, Oxford
53. Giora R (ed) (2007) Is metaphor special? Brain Lang 100:111-114
54. Roehm D, Bornkessel-Schlewiesky I, Roesler F, Schlewiesky M (2007) To predict or not to predict: influences of task and strategy on the processing of semantic relations. J Cogn Neurosci 19:1259-1274
55. Kutas M, Iragui V (1998) The N400 in a semantic categorization task across 6 decades. Electroencephalogr Clin Neurophysiol 108:456-471
56. Donchin E, Coles MGH (1988) Is the P300 component a manifestation of context updating? Behav Brain Sci 11:357-374
57. Picton TW (1993) The P300 wave of the human event-related brain potentials. J Clin Neurophysiol 9:456-479
58. Verleger R (1988) Event-related potentials and cognition: a critique of the context updating hypothesis and an alternative interpretation of P3. Behav Brain Sci 11:343-327.
59. Verleger R (1997) On the utility of the P3 latency as an index of mental chronometry. Psychophysiology 34:131-156
60. Kok A (2001) On the utility of P3 amplitude as a measure of processing capacity. Psychophysiology 38:557-577
61. Chao L, Nielsen-Bohlman LC, Knight RT (1995) Auditory even-related potentials dissociate early and late memory processes. Electroencephalogr Clin Neurophysiol 96:157-168
62. Rugg MD, Doyle MC (1992) Event-related potentials and recognition memory for low- and high-frequency words. J Cogn Neurisci 4:69-79
63. Bar M (2007) The proactive brain: using analogies and associations to generate predictions. Trends Cogn Sci 11:7:280-289

Towards a Neurophysiology of Language 8

S.F. Cappa

8.1 Introduction

Scientific study of the relationship between language and the human brain started in the second half of the nineteenth century, as one of the many aspects of experimental medicine, and, in particular, of experimental physiology [1]. There is no need to retell a story that has already been told several times (for an excellent, very readable review, see [2]). The specific limitation in the case of language was, of course, that experimental studies in animals are not possible. However, an answer to this obstacle came from clinical neurology, when several astute physicians, whose names form the Hall of Fame of neuropsychology, such as Broca and Wernicke, inaugurated systematic application of the anatomico-clinical method to the study of language disorders. The logic of this approach took advantage of those accidents of nature, i.e., spontaneously occurring brain lesions. Information gathered from observations of the clinical picture, combined with knowledge about the location of the lesion in the brain, allowed the "localization" of cognitive functions to discrete brain regions. In the case of language, this led to the development of the classical Wernicke-Lichtheim model of word processing, which still finds an honorable place in practically every textbook dealing with aphasia [3]. The model's fortunes and, in general, those of what Head called the "diagram-makers," have fluctuated over the years—with eclipses during the golden age of gestalt psychology and, sometime, later, by the advent of behaviorism [4]. What is important to underline here is that acceptance of the idea that complex aspects of language, such as syntax, or the lexicon, could be localized to specific brain areas has gone largely unchallenged well into the era of cognitive neuroscience. Experimental approaches have been expanded and supported by the advent

S.F. Cappa (✉)
Vita-Salute San Raffaele University and Division of Neuroscience, San Raffaele Scientific Institute, Milan, Italy

of functional imaging methods, in particular functional magnetic resonance imaging (fMRI) [5]. The aspects of language that have been localized often reflect, rather than the coarse definition of modalities of language use or of levels of linguistic organization, sophisticated psycholinguistic models [6]. The underlying anatomy is in general considered to parallel this complexity and is usually defined in terms of networks of brain regions, not specific areas. Nevertheless, a large part of this recent research shares with the traditional approach what Lord Brain, in a landmark paper, called "jumping from psychology to anatomy" [7], as it lacks any hypothesis about the physiological mechanisms responsible for the specific anatomical localization. Within this framework, for example, the cortex is considered as a more or less homogeneous structure, and an activation shown with fMRI simply represents a location in space, which for mysterious reasons is associated with a specific task [8]. It must be noted that, by comparison, early researchers, such as Wernicke and Freud, were much more ambitious, as they attempted to interpret the localizations within the physiological knowledge available at the time [9].

However, the situation has been rapidly changing and the criticisms frequently raised against the "correlative" information provided by fMRI studies have played an important role in stimulating new approaches to data analysis, going beyond the classical "cognitive subtraction" approach [10]. An important example is provided by methods that measure integration among brain areas [11]. In addition, a biological approach to language has been stimulated by generative linguistics [12] and the findings supported by discoveries in genetics [13, 14]. The definition of a "neurobiology of language" may at the moment sound overambitious, but reflects the effort to go beyond a mere correlation between a level of linguistic analysis and putative brain areas subserving the corresponding level of processing. Instead, the final aim is to investigate the neurophysiological mechanisms that may be responsible for specific components of linguistic function. In this chapter, I present a very selective review of those areas of neuroscience research on language that I consider to be particularly promising from this standpoint.

8.2 The Neurobiology of Syntax

Syntax is the central aspect of language. The ability to combine linguistic elements in an infinite number of sentences is a unique component of human cognition, and the investigation of its neurological underpinnings has long been a topic of neurolinguistic research. Most of the available evidence is derived from two lines of investigations: (1) the study of neurological patients who show defective syntactic production and comprehension, and (2) investigation of the brain correlates of syntactic processing in normal subjects by means of functional imaging or neurophysiological assessments. Both these areas of research have been recently reviewed (see, for example, [15, 16]). One original line of investigation is based on a study of the brain correlates of the acquisition of linguistic rules. A crucial aspect of language form this point of view is that some rules are not found in any human languages [17]. In particular, the linear order of words does not have a role in the establishment of syntactic dependencies in any language. The basic mechanism is hierarchical phrase structure, generated by recursive rules. A comparison of the neuroanatomical correlates underlying the acquisition of grammatical and non-grammatical rules shows that only the former specifically activate Broca's area. In one experiment, the subjects were asked to learn several rules of an artificial language that had been developed in order to identify the neural correlates of specific syntactic processing [18]. Grammatically possible rules were based on hierarchical syntactic notions, such as "the article always immediately follows the noun it refers to." Impossible rules were based on linear relationships, such as "the article always follows the second word in a sentence." The acquisition of the possible rules specifically activated a left hemispheric network, including Broca's area, as shown by direct comparisons between the two rule types. The selective role of Broca's area was further confirmed by time-condition interactions and by proficiency effects, in that higher proficiency in grammatical rule usage, but not in usage of non-grammatical rules, led to higher levels of activation in Broca's area [19]. Comparable results were obtained by teaching the subjects real languages [20]. German students were asked to learn real rules of Italian and Japanese, i.e., two very different languages, which they did not know, but which follow the principles of universal grammar (UG) [21]. In a contrast condition, they had to learn a different set of invented "rules," which were of comparable difficulty but violated the principles of UG, framed in the same lexical context (i.e., Italian or Japanese). These were of the form (for example): "in order to negate a sentence, insert the word "no" after the third word." This rule violates UG because no language includes rules based on the linear order of words. The students were able to master the real, as well as the unreal rules with comparable proficiency after the training session. However, the comparison of brain activity between the two conditions indicated that the improvement in performance was paralleled by an increased activation of Broca's area only in the case of real, hierarchical grammatical rules.

A recent study [22] extended this model, based on the hypothesis of a specific function of Broca's area in the acquisition and usage of recursive hierarchical rules, by contrasting the neural activity paralleling the acquisition by normal subjects of a "rigid" syntax, in which an element must occur at a fixed distance from another word, and of a non-rigid syntax, in which distances between elements are specified in terms of relative position and can always be recursively expanded. As underlined above, rules based on rigid distances, are never found in grammars of human languages. In this experiment, the rules were applied to sequences of non-linguistic, visual stimuli (Korean letters, totally unknown to the subjects). The results were formally compared with those of obtained in the previous experiment on the language domain [19] and indicated a largely overlapping pattern of results. Both in the visuo-spatial and in the language domain, the acquisition of non-rigid syntax, but not of rigid syntax, activated the Brodmann area 44 component of the Broca's region. This domain-independent effect was specifically modulated by performance improvement also in the case of visuo-spatial rule acquisition.

Taken together, these results address the crucial issue of the functional role of

8

Broca's area (see [23] for a complete overview of this brain region). They support the claim of its specialized role in the analysis, the recognition and prediction of non-linear structural relationships within linguistic and non-linguistic domains, including the executive control of hierarchically organized action sequences [24]. Brodmann area 44 in the monkey is responsible for the control of orofacial actions [25]. This is the area in which neurons with mirror properties (activated both by action execution and action observation) were originally recorded [26]. These and other observations have revived the debate about the relationship between language and the motor system [27-29]. While any effort to reduce the complex formal aspects of syntax, as described by generative linguistics, to the action system seems to be doomed to failure, this line of investigation may be fruitful in evaluating the possibility that a functional system dedicated to the representation of abstract hierarchical dependencies has developed from the neural mechanism of action control and action representation.

8.3 Semantic Representations in the Brain

Interest in the neurological basis of knowledge about entities, events, and words originates from the classical neuropsychological observations of visual agnosia and transcortical sensory aphasia, which provided direct evidence that brain damage can impair selected aspects of knowledge. In the last few decades, observations of patients with categorical knowledge disorders, in particular for living entities or artifacts, as well as the description of semantic dementia have attracted increasing attention to this topic. There are several competing cognitive theories about semantic memory organization. Symbolic theories propose an amodal organization of semantic memory but do not necessary entail predictions about the neural correlates of amodal knowledge. However, an important role of the anterior temporal lobe has been proposed on the basis of evidence from semantic dementia [30].

Recently, theories that ground knowledge in the perception and action systems of the brain (embodied, or grounded, cognition, [31]) have challenged this view. A precursor of this approach is certainly the work of Carl Wernicke. In 1874, he wrote, "The concept of the word "bell", for example, is formed by the associated memory images of visual, tactual and auditory perceptions. These memory images represent the essential characteristic features of the object, bell." [9]. In 1885: "Close association between these various memory images has been established by repeated experience of the essential features of bells. As a final result, arousal of each individual image is adequate for awakening the concept as a whole. In this way a functional unit is achieved. Such units form the concept of the object, in this case a bell." [32]. In 1900: "In the cortex we can again ascribe this role to certain cells: a transient stimulus can cause lasting modifications in these cells so that some form of residuum of the stimulus remains, which we call a memory trace. [...] These facts prove beyond any doubt that memory traces are localized to their respective projection fields" and "The important point is that associative processes can only be explained if we postulate functional interconnections among the anatomical regions to which the memory traces of the individual sensory modalities are localized." [33]. The idea that high-order cognitive processes are based on the partial reactivation of states in sensory, motor, and affective systems has a very long history in philosophy and psychology [34].

The general concept that the neural system underlying semantic knowledge is distributed in the brain is clearly supported by functional imaging studies. Most of these studies evidence dynamic maps of conceptual and lexical representations, which are modulated by task demands as well as by the type of knowledge and the modality of stimulus presentation (for a recent review, see [35]). While the engagement of regions related to perceptual and action processing during conceptual tasks is supported by most of the studies, the interpretation of the functional role of these activations remains open. In addition, several findings are compatible with the idea of an additional level of categorical organization, which can be considered as an emerging property (as proposed in [36]) or a superordinate principle that encompasses modality-specific activation [37]. A large number of investigations have addressed the neural mechanisms associated with the processing of words referring to a specific class of knowledge, i.e., action and movement. In particular, several studies have shown that listening to verbs related to actions performed by different body parts (mouth, hand, or foot) activates, besides the classical language areas, brain regions associated with actions actually performed with the same body parts [38, 39] (Fig. 8.1).

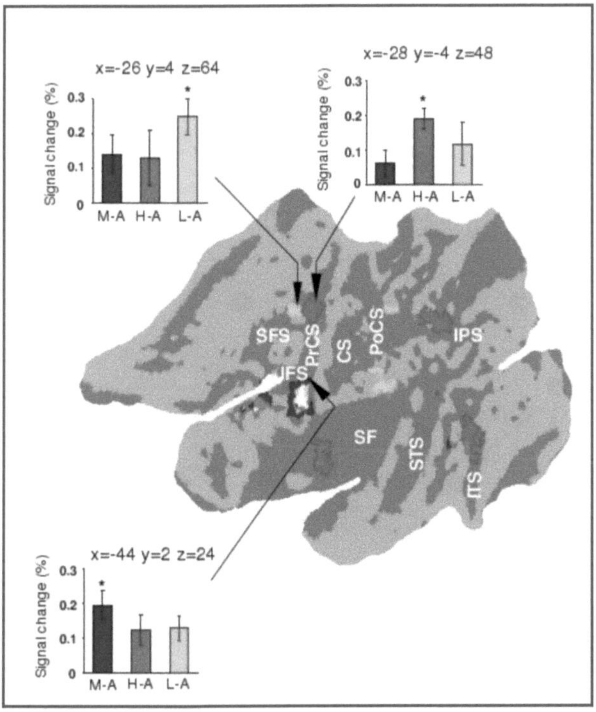

Fig. 8.1 Areas activated by action sentences referring to different body parts (comparison with comparable abstract sentences) represented on a "flattened" brain. *M-A,* mouth action; *H-A,* hand action; *L-A,* leg actions; *SFS,* superior frontal sulcus; *IFS,* inferior frontal sulcus; *PrCS,* precentral sulcus; *CS,* central sulcus; *PostCS,* posterior central sulcus; *SF,* Sylvian fissure; *STS,* superior temporal sulcus; *ITS,* inferior temporal sulcus; *IPS,* inferior parietal sulcus

A recent experiment has added relevant information about the possible functional role of these activations. The study is basically replicates a previous investigation [39], in which subjects were simply asked to listen to transitive sentences, which could refer to action ("I push the button") or to abstract ("I appreciate the loyalty") concepts, with the addition of sentences, including sentential negation, i.e., a universal syntactic feature of human languages that reverses the truth value expressed by a sentence. The comparison between affirmative and negative sentences indicated that the presence of sentential negation was, overall, associated with a decreased activation of both several cortical regions and a subcortical structure, the left pallidum. As in the previous experiment, action-related sentences, as opposed to abstract sentences, activated the left-hemispheric action-representation system. Specifically, the activity within the action-representation system was reduced for negative action-related *vs* affirmative action-related sentences (compared to abstract sentences). The analysis of functional integration within the cerebral areas forming the action system, as measured by dynamic causal modeling, was weaker for negative action-related than for affirmative action-related sentences (Fig. 8.2).

These findings suggest that sentential negation transiently reduces the access to mental representations of the negated information [40], and provide additional evidence for a link between the action system and language representation at the semantic level.

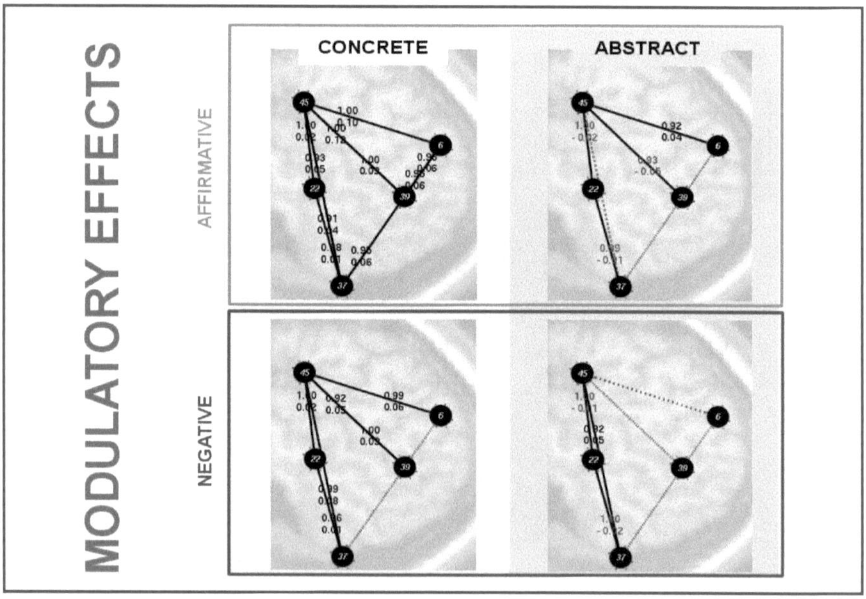

Fig. 8.2 Results of dynamic causal modeling analysis of functional integration among brain regions (numbers refer to Brodmann's areas)

8.4
Multiple Pathways for Language Processing

The role of white-matter pathways in language processing is a classic tenet of aphasiology, from the writings of Carl Wernicke [9] to the disconnection account of neuropsychological syndromes resurrected by Norman Geschwind in the 1960s [41]. In the last few years, the possibility to visualize white-matter pathways in vivo, using diffusion tensor imaging (DTI) and tractography, has led to renewed interest in the concept of functional disconnection [42]. In the case of language, one interesting development originated from the proposal of extension of the dual-pathways model from vision to audition. The distinction between a ventral, occipito-temporal pathway dedicated to object recognition ("what"), and a dorsal, occipito-parietal pathway responsible for object localization [43] has been extremely influential in neuropsychology. For example, a different, but related proposal based on the distinction between a ventral "perception" pathway and a dorsal "action" pathway has led to crucial insights in visuo-perceptual disorders due to cortical lesions [44]. The application of a similar framework to auditory perception is to the result of the work of one of the leading figures in auditory neurophysiology, Josef Rauschenker [45], and had an immediate impact on the neurobiology of language. In the classical textbook model of Wernicke-Lichtheim, the area of "auditory images" in the left temporal lobe is connected, via a single fiber tract, the arcuate fasciculus, to Broca's area in the prefrontal lobe. Recent models of language processing, which have been developed, in particular, on the basis of functional imaging investigations of speech perception and speech production, have attempted to integrate the neurophysiological concept of dual auditory pathways within multiple network models of language organization in the brain. The ventral auditory pathway in non-human primates plays a crucial role in auditory object recognition, connecting the anterior auditory regions to the ventrolateral prefrontal cortex. The dorsal pathway is specialized for auditory spatial localization, and connects the caudal belt area to the dorsolateral prefrontal cortex [46]. Can this model be extended to human brains, in which audition has differentiated to become the main modality subserving language use? Several different proposals are based on the distinction between a dorsal and a ventral language pathway. A crucial step in this direction is the identification of two separate anterior-posterior networks of areas connected by specific fiber tracts. The proposal of a ventral pathway is supported by a number of independent sources of evidence. In the first place, many functional imaging studies of speech perception have indicated a separation in the associative auditory areas between an anterior stream (anterior superior temporal gyrus, middle temporal gyrus, superior temporal sulcus) and a posterior stream, corresponding to the planum temporale and the temporo-parietal junction (i.e., the traditional "Wernicke's area") [47]. The anterior stream is specifically activated by intelligible speech, and is responsible for language comprehension [48]. The second line of evidence for a crucial role of the anterior temporal lobe in language comprehension and, in general, in semantic processing was provided by the investigation of patients with semantic dementia, in which this part of the brain is affected early and severely [30].

The third important element for the delineation of a ventral pathway is the identification of long fiber connections reaching the frontal lobe. It is noteworthy that Wernicke, in his original formulation of a pathway account of language physiology, suggested that the connection between anterior and posterior language areas was provided by the insula and the underlying white matter [49]. Recent magnetic resonance tractography studies have indicated the existence of a ventral route, located in the region of the external [50] or extreme capsule [49], thus supporting Wernicke's original intuition.

Within this renewed framework, the classical route from temporal to frontal lobe through the arcuate fasciculus is a reasonable candidate for the dorsal pathway in humans. In this case, application of the neurophysiological label the "where" pathway is not as straightforward as in the case of the ventral "what" pathway. It is actually the alternate concept of an action-related function [44] that can be mapped to the concept of sensorimotor transformation necessary for speech production. One proposal is that the posterior auditory regions are responsible for matching incoming auditory information with stored templates, thus constraining speech production [51]. Recently [46], a specific computational role was proposed for the dorsal processing stream, in which a key role is played by the inferior parietal lobule (IPL). According to this model, the IPL receives an efference copy of articulatory plans from Broca's area, as well as a fast sketch of sensory events from the posterior auditory areas, allowing real-time control through a continuous comparison of intended and ongoing speech production.

Additional, relevant information was provided by the studies of Friederici's group [52], which found an anatomical fractionation within Broca's region—with a deep region activated by the computation of local (non-hierarchical) dependencies—and Broca's area proper that was selectively engaged by hierarchical dependencies (see above). Tractographic studies with DTI indicated that the two regions have distinct fiber projections: the deep opercular region to the anterior temporal lobe via the uncinate fasciculus, and Broca's area proper via the arcuate fasciculus to the posterior perisylvian region [53]. The deep frontal operculum-anterior temporal lobe system in this model is responsible for local phrase-structure building. The second, dorsal system, which includes Broca's area proper, is responsible for the computation of long-distance dependencies engaging working memory resources, and includes the posterior superior temporal gyrus, responsible for final sentence integration.

8.5 Conclusions

One of the early concerns about the application of functional imaging methods to investigations of the neural basis of cognitive functions was centered on the idea that the results provided by the new tools mostly confirmed classical notions derived by anatomico-clinical observations in neurological patients. The development of cognitive neuroscience research in the last decade has certainly challenged this prediction.

Functional imaging, comprising a continuously improving array of methodologies allowing in vivo explorations of brain activity in the spatial and temporal domains, is now generating new hypotheses about the neural foundation of cognitive functions. Language is no exception, and the selected examples presented in this chapter represent promising forays into its neurobiological underpinnings.

References

1. Finger S (1994) Origins of neuroscience. Oxford University Press, New York
2. Shorto R (2008) Descartes' bones: a skeletal history of the conflict between faith and reason. Doubleday, New York
3. Poeppel D, Hickok G (2004) Towards a new functional anatomy of language. Cognition 92:1-12
4. Cappa SF (2007) Linguaggio. In: Gallese V (ed) Dizionario storico delle Neuroscienze. Einaudi, Torino
5. Demonet JF, Thierry G, Cardebat D (2005) Renewal of the neurophysiology of language: functional neuroimaging. Physiol Rev 85:49-95
6. Indefrey P, Levelt P (2000) The neural correlates of language production. In: Gazzaniga MS (ed) The new cognitive neurosciences. The MIT Press, Cambridge
7. Brain R (1961) The neurology of language. Brain 84:145-166
8. Legrenzi P, Umiltà C (2008) Neuromania. Il Mulino, Bologna.
9. Wernicke C (1874) Der aphasische Symptomencomplex. Cohn und Weigert, Breslau
10 Friston KJ, Price CJ, Fletcher P et al (1996) The trouble with cognitive subtraction. Neuroimage 4:97-104
11. Penny WD, Stephan KE, Mechelli A, Friston KJ (2004) Modelling functional integration: a comparison of structural equation and dynamic causal models. Neuroimage 23 Suppl 1:S264-274
12. Fitch WT, Hauser MD, Chomsky N (2005) The evolution of the language faculty: clarifications and implications. Cognition 97:179-210; discussion 211-125
13. Abrahams BS, Tentler D, Perederiy JV et al (2007) Genome-wide analyses of human perisylvian cerebral cortical patterning. Proc Natl Acad Sci USA 104:17849-17854
14. White SA, Fisher SE, Geschwind DH et al (2006) Singing mice, songbirds, and more: models for FOXP2 function and dysfunction in human speech and language. J Neurosci 26:10376-10379
15. Grodzinsky Y, Friederici AD (2006) Neuroimaging of syntax and syntactic processing. Curr Opin Neurobiol 16:240-246
16. Moro A (2008) The boundaries of Babel. The brain and the enigma of impossible languages. MIT Press, Cambridge, MA
17. Moro A, Tettamanti M, Perani D et al (2001) Syntax and the brain: disentangling grammar by selective anomalies. Neuroimage 13:110-118
18. Tettamanti M, Alkadhi H, Moro A et al (2002) Neural correlates for the acquisition of natural language syntax. Neuroimage 17:700-709.
19. Musso M, Moro A, Glauche V et al (2003) Broca's area and the language instinct. Nat Neurosci 6:774-781
20. Chomsky N (1986) Knowledge of language: its nature, origin and use. Praeger, New York
21. Tettamanti M, Rotondi I, Perani D et al (2009) Syntax without language: neurobiological evidence for cross-domain syntactic computations. Cortex 45:825-838
22. Grodzinsky Y, Amunts K (2006) The Broca's region. Oxford University Press, New York

8

23. Koechlin E, Ody C, Kouneiher F (2003) The architecture of cognitive control in the human prefrontal cortex. Science 302:1181-1185
24. Petrides M, Cadoret G, Mackey S (2005) Orofacial somatomotor responses in the macaque monkey homologue of Broca's area. Nature 435:1235-1238
25. Rizzolatti G, Craighero L (2004) The mirror-neuron system. Annu Rev Neurosci 27:169-192
26. Rizzolatti G, Arbib MA (1998) Language within our grasp. Trends Neurosci 21:188-194
27. Pulvermuller F (2005) Brain mechanisms linking language and action. Nat Rev Neurosci 6:576-582
28. Fazio P, Cantagallo A, Craighero L et al (2009) Encoding of human action in Broca's area. Brain 132:1980-1988
29. Patterson K, Nestor PJ, Rogers TT (2007) Where do you know what you know? The representation of semantic knowledge in the human brain. Nat Rev Neurosci 8:976-988
30. Barsalou LW (2008) Grounded cognition. Annu Rev Psychol 59:617-645
31. Wernicke C (1885-1886/1977) Einige neuere Arbeiten ueber Aphasie. In: Eggert GH (ed) Wernicke's works on aphasia: a sourcebook and review. Mouton, The Hague
32. Wernicke C (1900) Grundriss der Psychiatrie. Thieme, Leipzig
33. Prinz JJ (2002) Furnishing the mind: concepts and their perceptual basis. MIT Press, Cambridge, MA
34. Cappa SF (2008) Imaging studies of semantic memory. Curr Opin Neurol 21:669-675
35. Martin A (2007) The representation of object concepts in the brain. Annu Rev Psychol 58:25-45
36. Mahon BZ, Caramazza A (2008) A critical look at the embodied cognition hypothesis and a new proposal for grounding conceptual content. J Physiol Paris 102:59-70
37. Hauk O, Johnsrude I, Pulvermuller F (2004) Somatotopic representation of action words in human motor and premotor cortex. Neuron 41:301-307
38. Tettamanti M, Buccino G, Saccuman MC et al (2005) Listening to action-related sentences activates fronto-parietal motor circuits. J Cogn Neurosci 17:273-281
39. Tettamanti M, Manenti R, Della Rosa PA et al (2008) Negation in the brain: modulating action representations. Neuroimage 43:358-367
40. Geschwind N, Kaplan E (1962) A human cerebral disconnection syndrome. A preliminary report. Neurology 12:65-75
41. Catani M, ffytche DH (2005) The rises and falls of disconnection syndromes. Brain 128:2224-2239
42. Ungerleider LG, Mishkin M (1982) Two cortical visual systems. In: Dingle DJ (ed) Analysis of visual behavior. MIT Press, Cambridge, MA
43. Goodale MA, Milner AD (1992) Separate visual pathways for perception and action. Trends Neurosci 15:20-25
44. Rauschecker JP, Tian B (2000) Mechanisms and streams for processing of "what" and "where" in auditory cortex. Proc Nat Acad Sci USA 97:11800-11806
45. Rauschecker JP, Scott SK (2009) Maps and streams in the auditory cortex: nonhuman primates illuminate human speech processing. Nat Neurosci 12:718-724
46. Wise RJS (2003) Language systems in normal and aphasic human subjects: functional imaging studies and inferences from animal studies. Brit Med Bull 65:95-119
47. Scott SK, Blank CC, Rosen S, Wise RJ (2000) Identification of a pathway for intelligible speech in the left temporal lobe. Brain 123:2400-2406
48. Saur D, Schelter B, Schnell S, Kratochvil D et al (2010) Combining functional and anatomical connectivity reveals brain networks for auditory language comprehension. Neuroimage 49: 3187-3197
49. Parker GJ, Luzzi S, Alexander DC et al (2005) Lateralization of ventral and dorsal auditory-language pathways in the human brain. Neuroimage 24:656-666

50. Saur D, Kreher BW, Schnell S et al (2008) Ventral and dorsal pathways for language. Proc Natl Acad Sci USA 105:18035-18040
51. Warren JE, Wise RJ, Warren JD (2005) Sounds do-able: auditory-motor transformations and the posterior temporal plane. Trends Neurosci 28:636-643
52. Friederici AD, Bahlmann J, Heim S et al (2006) The brain differentiates human and non-human grammars: functional localization and structural connectivity. Proc Natl Acad Sci USA 103:2458-2463
53. Anwander A, Tittgemeyer M, von Cramon DY et al (2006) Connectivity-based parcellation of Broca's area. Cereb Cortex 17:816-825

Section III
From Intentions to Nonverbal Communication

Intentions and Communication: Cognitive Strategies, Metacognition and Social Cognition

9

M. Balconi

9.1
Introduction: Communication as an Intentionalization Process

Communicating involves different complex processes. A prerequisite of communication is the intentional planning of the entire process, that is, the conscious selection of meanings, adequate behavioral strategies, and communicative goals. In particular, we define an intentionalization process as a dynamic operation that actively involves speaker and listener: the former is engaged in the formulation and expression of his or her own intention to produce an effect on the listener (*intentionalization*); the listener, in turn, needs to interpret the speaker's communicative intention (*re-intentionalization*) [1-3]. An intentionalization process consists of a number of functions that allow the communicative process to take place: the definition of *communicative goals*; the establishment of *behavioral strategies* for communication performance; the *monitoring* and *self-monitoring* of the communicative process; and the feedback produced by the interlocutor. The entire system makes use of a set of coordination competences that are essential to the regulation of intentions. In particular, the articulation of intentional systems requires the activity of attentional mechanisms aiming, on the one hand, to select information and to produce appropriate representations (*representational communicative level*), and, on the other hand, to organize the enactor system (*communicative actions planning*). Those operations implicate the activity of *central coordination mechanisms*, intended as the meta-level-controlled processes that require the speaker's voluntary and conscious actions [4]. In this chapter, we first focus on the relationship between intentionality and communicative intentions, highlighting the role of consciousness in communication. Second, we consider the role of attention in control operations. Finally, we discuss action planning,

M. Balconi (✉)
Department of Psychology, Catholic University of Milan, Milan, Italy

Neuropsychology of Communication. Michela Balconi (Ed.)

strategy definition, and the monitoring and self-monitoring of communication outcomes and effects.

9.1.1 Intentionality and Communicative Intention

Intentionality can be defined as the mental condition of being oriented toward something, and intentional action as the representation of a goal, implying the ability to deliberately differentiate means and aims [5, 6]. This definition of intentionality includes some important properties: intention direction (*being oriented towards*), mental/representational dimension (*having a representation of*), and psychological value (*being aimed at*). Moreover, in order to formulate an intention, it is necessary to distinguish between the self (internal world) and the external world; this distinction constitutes the interactive and relational component of intention (*intentional relations*). In fact, intentional activity is always performed by an agent and it is aimed toward something or somebody perceived as external [7].

Nonetheless, intention is not an all-or-nothing concept: instead, it is possible to distinguish different degrees of intentionality, ranging from focused attention on external stimuli or internal mental states and actions to automatic responses to internal or external stimuli. From an ontogenetic perspective, there is a noteworthy coincidence between the development of cognitive abilities and the acquisition of control functions for the intentional regulation of action plans. In fact, motor action shows a clear organization, in terms of a clear means-goals distinction, throughout individual development and this acquisition parallels the acquisition of cognitive competence aimed at the representation of mental states (*meta-cognition*) [8, 9].

Intentional action can be distinguished from non-intentional action by referring to two interrelated concepts: *consciousness* and *attention*. Thus, both the awareness of one's own behavior and the intentional regulation of actions become flexible and discriminative elements as a function of the action's global aims.

On the communicative level, the modulation of intentions characterizes communication flow, from minimum conditions of intentionality (*automatic communicative actions*, such as waving to greet someone) to maximum conditions of intentionality (*meta-intentional communicative actions*, e.g., to lie). The latter are characterized by high cognitive complexity and require the joint intervention of attentional functions and consciousness as fundamental mechanisms in the intentional and strategic planning of communicative action.

9.1.2 Intention and Consciousness

Consciousness has been described as: (1) *perceptual, cognitive and meta-cognitive awareness*, (2) a *high-order cognitive faculty*, or (3) as a *conscious state* as opposed to an unconscious one [10]. Here, we define consciousness as a set of properties necessary for the cognitive awareness of one's own choices. It is, therefore, a meta-process that is involved in determining courses of action and which presides over mnestic functions. Moreover, consciousness can be defined by a limited number of abilities and characterized by a variable degree of intentionality [11].

A peculiar element of consciousness is the paradox of wholeness through multiplicity: consciousness unitarity is the result of different processes operating simultaneously (*wholeness*). But it is also defined by a multiplicity of components at the level of content; in other words, consciousness is the result of the functional convergence of a number of complex informative systems (*multiplicity*) [12]. This conception is supported on the anatomic level by the "distributed" nature of consciousness, as evidenced by the simultaneous activation of different neural systems during conscious mental operations. In particular, the *distributed processual model* stresses the necessity of the distributed nature of structural systems supporting consciousness, since different functions comprise that process. According to this model, consciousness can be defined as: (a) a system involved in the integration of computational units; (b) a system that allows an increase in the activity within a specific neural system, in order to perform specific cognitive functions. These properties do not require convergent information to be placed within a single anatomic structure; rather they demand that the structure supporting consciousness is able to integrate information coming from anatomically separated systems. Therefore, consciousness can be seen as a distributed neural network involving the different neural activities underlying the conscious experience.

9.1.3 Consciousness and Attention: Two Autonomous Systems

How is it possible to define consciousness's specific role in intentional communication planning? In order to understand consciousness with respect to communicative intentionalization processes, it is necessary to acknowledge the distinction between aware and unaware processes. The distinction is based on the differentiation of involved cognitive processes, on the way information is organized, and on the attentional level and cognitive effort required [13]. These properties, however, do not seem to be exclusive to conscious processes, rather they characterize unconscious processes as well. For instance, during subliminal stimulation, a stimulus is not consciously elaborated by the subject, although it remains present in active information selection [14]; this operation involves finalized orientation and the ability to elaborate stimuli features. Rather, the conscious/unconscious distinction refers to the relationships that conscious contents may establish with other active cognitive processes. Specifically, the *integrated field model* [15] suggests that the exceptional property of conscious processes is their contextuality, i.e., the relation that conscious contents establish with other contents/processes within the elaboration system. In fact, although sensorial input, elaborated outside consciousness fields, might modify the probability that a specific behavior occurs, the process appears to be independent from any other individual's condition or mental state, such that data cannot be encoded within the memory system.

9

An additional issue is whether consciousness is involved only in attentional controlled processes or also in automatic processes. In the latter case, consciousness would completely coincide with attentional functions. However, it might be possible that consciousness operates also within automatic processes, albeit to different degrees. In fact, consciousness functions may indirectly exercise control over automatic mechanisms, determining the conscious goals to be fulfilled. In addition, consciousness might exercise direct control over controlled processes, organizing executive sequences of mental operations. For these reasons, the *independency model* [16] suggests that consciousness and attention are dissociated systems. This model is based on the existence of attentional processes that do not involve consciousness (as when driving a car, in which case we pay attention without actually being conscious of it), and of objects/stimuli that we might become conscious of without paying attention to them (as in dichotic listening, in which in the absence of attention an unusual stimulus might reach our consciousness). The double dissociation between attention-mediated operations and consciousness makes plausible the existence of two autonomous systems that interact with one another.

On the anatomico-structural level, empirical evidence endorses the existence of two independent systems [17, 18]. Moreover, the development of both faculties presided over by consciousness and attentional processes supports a clear temporal dissociation: general attentional functions seem to develop earlier, while the ability to coordinate and plan intentional actions appears around nine months of age. This acquisition implies the development of the mind; specifically, the ability to represent one's self and others, which is a necessary condition for the formulation of a theory of mind, as well as the ability to intentionally organize and plan courses of action [19].

Generally, as opposed to the attentional system, which is only involved in action selection, consciousness is also involved in the selection of thoughts, since it provides the basis for voluntary action and is fundamental in the active choice of specific courses of actions within specific communicative contexts.

9.1.4 Consciousness Functions for Communication

What are the specific functions of consciousness for communication regulation? First, consciousness allows control of priority information access. Examples of this mechanism are the selection and control functions of representational components destined to become part of consciousness. Through the selection of priorities, in fact, it is possible to define information access criteria. The passage of certain contents to the conscious system allows the organism's adaptation to the environment, on the basis of its needs and of the communication goals [20]. Furthermore, consciousness operates to respond to the flexibility requirements of knowledge organization. More generally, a thinking system needs to be involved in the optimization of its processes, alternating rigid and automatic response structures with flexible modalities. The latter are useful in new, unpredictable situations, in which consolidated automatic responses are not adequate. On a further level, consciousness directly intervenes in the activation of mental and physical actions and in the regulation of executive functions for decision-making (see Par. 9.2). An example of this is provided by the definition of conscious aims for the organization of motor systems involved in voluntary non-verbal communicative actions. Finally, consciousness is involved in higher-order cognitive functions of self-monitoring and reflexive functions (see Par. 9.3).

Globally, consciousness grants access to multiple and independent representational sources. Coherent information organization and control functions of intentional action appear to have priority in the first phases of consciousness-communication regulation, while self-monitoring and reflexive function allow a progressive adaptation to the interactive communication context. Consciousness therefore makes a relevant contribution to the flexible management of knowledge and to the configuration of multiple systems specialized in self-representation: the awareness of one's own actions and the re-calibration of actions become discriminative elements [21]. Figure 9.1 summarizes the principal functions of consciousness for the planning of action and communication, in relation to the different levels involved.

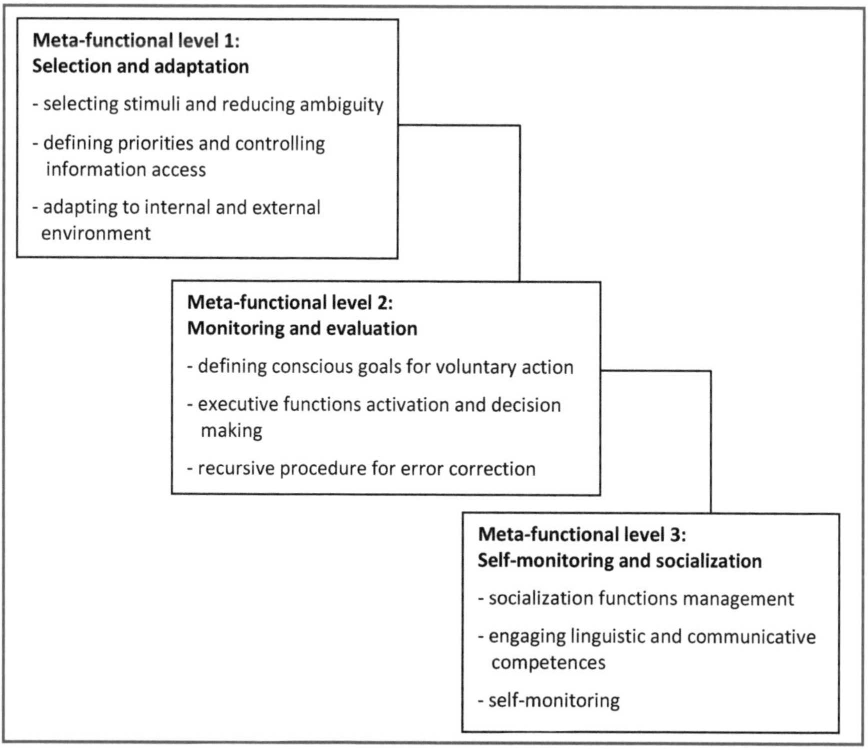

Fig. 9.1 Representation of the functions and levels of consciousness, especially, action planning and monitoring functions

9

9.2 Planning and Control of Communicative Action

9.2.1 Executive Functions

It is also important to identify the role and contribution of attentional systems and memory functions (in particular, working memory) to the definition of intentional action for communication. First of all, we need to introduce a system that is not directly implicated in cognitive state representation but instead serves to organize and co-ordinate mental functions, in order to fulfil communicative goals. These *executive functions* are able to interpret operations executed under attentional control.

Among the different models, we consider the one proposed by Shallice [22], which highlights three major executive functions: attentive orientation, discrimination, and alert system conservation. In particular, discrimination is the executive unit that includes awareness, semantic elaboration, and the intentional allocation of attentional resources. Moreover, the model predicts the existence of a central control system, separated from the peripheral processes that are under its control. This central system maintains representational and strategic competences but requires attentional resources and intentional effort since it possesses limited elaboration ability and cognitive resources. Globally, Shallice's model predicts the co-presence of two different systems for behavioral regulation. The first consists of a cognitive system for the automatic processing of information and intentional behavior regulation. This *competitive selection system* (CSS) functions to automatically activate a sequence of actions/behaviors without requiring attentional resources, as long as inhibitory processes intervene to end it. The second, *supervisory attentional system* (SAS) requires the allocation of attentional resources for conscious decision-making processes. SAS is active only under specific conditions, such as when no automatic schemes from the CSS are available, or during the performance of complex tasks, when subjective direct control is necessary.

Regarding the communicative level, the attentional control system is thought to have access to a complete representation of the external world and the individual's intentions, while, at the same time, it operates as a strategic system that determines and orients communicative choices within a specific context. Thus, it allows the representation of action/planning hierarchies by wielding attentional control over selection mechanisms, modulating the attentional level of the different operations. The intervention of automatic or controlled processes is calibrated in time. In fact, the existence of internal or external complex cognitive and emotional factors requires the contribution of an intentional decision mechanism, notwithstanding a greater use of cognitive resources than is the case under automatic conditions.

A number of studies have detected the partial or total inactivation of SAS control functions in patients with frontal lobe damages, accompanied by deficits in voluntary planning. These functions are replaced by the automatic functions of the CSS. Lesions to frontal areas may entail compromise of intentional coordination, strategic planning management, and general behavioral flexibility or the ability to program actions. Moreover, the lack of SAS functions entails direct manipulation of the subject's behavior by the external environment. In other words, individuals with SAS deficits tend to activate specific automatic behavioral schemes without the possibility to control actions.

9.2.2 Executive Functions for Intentional Communication

The relationship between executive functions and communication is complex. On the one hand, operations controlled by the executive system deal with functions of communicative act representation, i.e., as finalized action. On the other, these operations are directly involved in action execution planning and control. Accordingly, executive functions become a relevant factor for action supervision, directly affecting the communicative process. Those functions are intended as a set of processes aimed at regulating and directing behavior, through the management of super-ordinate operations such as the definition of strategies and plans, action hierarchies, and sequence organization, as well as the adaptation of a given strategy to context.

We now analyze the application of central control functions to communicative action planning, monitoring, and evaluation, from a cognitive and neuropsychological perspective. Intentional action planning requires a set of competencies presided over by central functions, such as the ability to *plan the action* as a function of a specific goal, to *flexibly use communicative strategies,* to *activate inferential processes*, and to *implement complex behaviors*. From the anatomico-structural perspective, specific areas (frontal and prefrontal cortex) constitute the anatomic substrate of executive functions, as reported in studies on lesions to anterior cerebral regions. These analyses evidenced a factual inability to plan, perform, and organize finalized actions in anterior-brain-damaged subjects. The frontal lobes, located frontally to the central sulcus, may be divided into four major areas: motor area, pre-motor area, prefrontal area, and the basomedial portion of the lobes. The last two are generally referred to as the prefrontal areas and they preside over higher cognitive faculties, including mnestic functions, reasoning, and intentional action. Support of superior processes is granted, on the anatomic level, based on the high number of connections with other cortical and subcortical areas, such as the basal ganglia and thalamus [23].

In particular, individuals reporting frontal deficits are characterized by a lack of flexible adaptation of communicative strategies and choices, and by a general difficulty in switching from one cognitive hypothesis to another. Those subjects show a prevalence of incorrect responses, even when provided with relevant feedbacks useful for error detection (*perseverance of erroneous behavior*). Individuals with executive deficits are also unable to use relevant information in order to predict behavioral outcomes or to evaluate particular situations (*deficits of cognitive evaluation*). The inability to formulate complex action plans involves different cognitive functions, such as hierarchical sequence organization, that define action execution priority. Deficits in global action sequence organization have been reported in subjects with frontal lesions, who show a global inability to organize intentional behavior (*deficits of sequence organization*). However, it is necessary to take note of the fact that the system that regulates executive function and the system that coordinates communicative processes appear to be different and to be characterized by autonomous mechanisms. In fact, deficits in the central executive system do not imply concomitant deficits in language representation abilities, as the former instead involves intentional planning functions. Aphasic individuals, with or without lesions to the left prefrontal dorso-lateral region, do not show differences in linguistic performance; however, subjects with extended lesions seem to have greater deficits in controlled actions execution [24].

9.2.3
Working Memory Contribution

An important role in the intentional regulation of linguistic tasks is played by the working memory system [25], comprising the central executive system, which is modality-dependent, and supportive components, such as the *phonological loop* and *visuo-spatial sketchpad*. Besides the control functions attributable to the central executive system, working memory is directly involved in linguistic and communicative processes, such as linguistic production and comprehension, and vocabulary acquisition. Recent models [26] suggest that working memory makes use of a storage system for the consolidation of semantic and syntactic information as well as phonological components. Working memory's contribution to representational processes, through specialized buffers, would require lower processes (storage, which can provide access to different representational formats) as well as superior ones (central executive). In particular, the contribution of phonological circuits appears to be fundamental in meaning comprehension, since it is active in the representation of linguistic inputs, as shown by the association between focal lesions to the phonological circuit and the ability to represent the meaning of words [27].

Selective deficits to working memory likely affect language comprehension. Here, we focus on the relation between phonological loop dysfunctions and sentence comprehension deficits. Patients with phonological loop deficits perform poorly in verbal-auditory string recall (numbers, letters, words). Some patients show deficits in short-term memory related to phonological storage [28], while in others deficits in rehearsal are seen [29]. These data support a connection between phonological deficits and language comprehension. It is possible to interpret this connection by concluding that phonological storage is necessary to support the initial phases of language comprehension, in which individuals operate a superficial sentence parsing when decoding appears to be particularly difficult. Comprehension difficulties related to complex sentences (characterized by semantic inversions or the presence of many closed-class words) have been detected in subjects with short-term memory deficits [30]. Phonological storage may be considered as a mnestic window [28] that maintains word order through phonological verbatim. A second explanation involves the role of phonological memory in second-level sentence analysis (after parsing and before sentence wrap-up), relative to post-syntactic thematic analysis [31, 32]. Finally, it is possible to assume a relationship between certain linguistic components and the phonological loop, and therefore a direct relation between linguistic task and phonological, syntactic, or semantic components. For instance, during a verbal recall task, syntactic and lexical components may be connected to phonological information. This model differs from the one proposed by Baddeley, in which working memory was not connected to any specific cognitive system. That model predicted the existence of specialized storage for semantic and syntactic information [33].

9.3 Action Strategies for Communication

Among the higher executive functions involved in communication, *strategic planning*, *monitoring*, and *self-monitoring* require specific cognitive competences. Those operations, in fact, imply the subject's ability to program actions following strategic aims, to evaluate the outcomes of these actions and to compare them with initial hypotheses, and, finally, to represent complex variables constituting communicative situations. Therefore, individuals must avail themselves of communication strategic planning on the one hand and meta-cognitive processes on the other. Both competencies retain a strong social valence and are involved in the entire communicative process, from initial planning to feedback analysis, finalized to subsequent interaction accommodation [34, 35].

9.3.1 Action Hierarchy Model

According to the action hierarchy model proposed by Stuss and Benson [36], behavioral control is performed through a hierarchical process (Fig. 9.2). At a lower level, perceptual information is elaborated through automatic processes, without conscious control. Brain posterior regions constitute the basis of these *elementary processes* in relation to the specific sensorial process involved (e.g., occipital areas for visual stimuli, temporal regions for auditory stimuli). A second level is associated with *supervisory executive functions*, related to the frontal lobe. This level is characterized by action anticipation, goal selection, planning and monitoring. The third level concerns *auto-reflexive functions*, which allows an individual to develop consciousness regarding his or her intentional choices and to access one's own cognitive processes (meta-cognition). In particular, auto-reflexive functions allow us to consciously regulate our relation to the external environment. This last level presides over the formulation of abstract representation used to select actions and the formulation of a global map of one's own cognitive behavior and that of other individuals as well as the regulation of meta-cognitive functions.

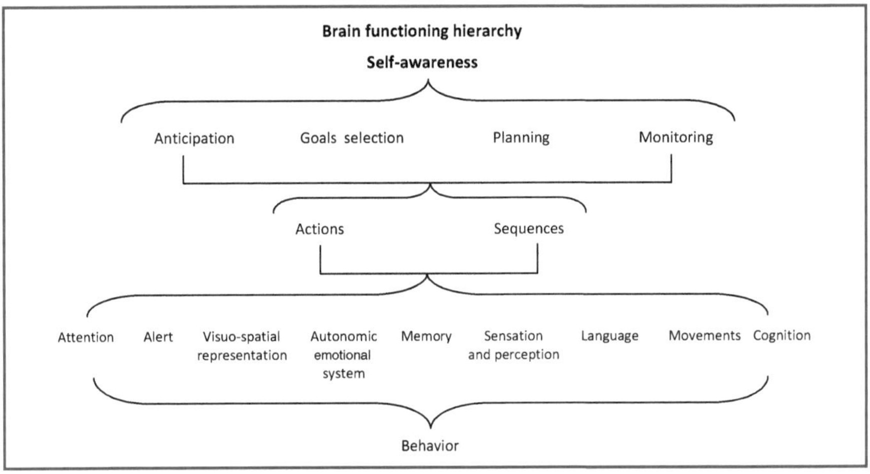

Fig. 9.2 Relation among behavioral systems, action mechanisms and consciousness mediation (self-awareness) in communicative behavior production

9.3.2
Strategy Implementation

The preceding discussion focused on strategic planning and action representation as two complex processes that involve a number of cognitive competences, such as the definition of a plan, which includes selecting action sequences, giving priorities to specific actions within action hierarchies, formulating outcome predictions and hypotheses related to the interactive context, and being able to flexibly adapt communicative strategies as a function of situational feedbacks. Here, we specifically analyze the anatomic components allowing general action strategy, the representation of schematic planning of action, and action preparation. These are considered as sequential phases, even if they are not necessarily distinguished on a temporal level.

9.3.2.1
Definition of Action Strategies

The definition of action strategies requires the contribution of different tasks organized in a sequential and functional order. The generation of strategic plans for intentional action presupposes the formulation of a global goal. This operation requires, in turn, the ability to use informative elements provided by the context in order to formulate an adequate course of action. In the next step, it is necessary to evaluate and predict possible action outcomes and to eventually modulate and change the plan according to contextual modifications. On an analytic level, strategic planning requires the selection of a sequence of actions that are appropriate for fulfilling specific goals and the continuous coordination of actions throughout the interaction.

9.3.2.2
Representation of a Schematic Planning of Action

The definition of a strategic action plan requires the more general competence of script generation. This competence is implied in our ability to plan, define actions and conceptualize situations, even when they are complex and articulated. At this point it is necessary to discuss the complex architecture underlying knowledge representation. The concept of script refers to a network of linked concepts, events, or actions all of which represent a global information unit comprising a heterogeneous number of informative elements. At the same time, scripts can be broken down into micro-analytic subcomponents, articulated on different cognitive levels.

The ability to store complex memory units with thematic (information and operations) and temporal (sequences) properties constitutes an advantage for the cognitive system, as evidenced by human evolution: thematic memory units are, in fact, stored in the pre-frontal cortex, which is more developed in humans than in any other species, thus explaining the unique abilities of the human mind with respect to goal-directed behavior. Moreover, on the ontogenetic level, the maturation of prefrontal areas appears to take more time (achieved at around 15 years of age) than is the case for the associative cortex. Thus, in the production and comprehension of schematic knowledge or complex events, this explains the individual's progressive passage from simple representational models to more complex models.

9.3.2.3
Action Preparation

The concept of action preparation involves *finalized behavior* and *motor preparation*. The former requires the selection of stimuli from the environmental information flow and the evaluation of their meanings. Finalized behavior has an adaptive role in strategic choice, since it involves coordination and mediation between internal needs (individual) and external demands (contextual). The concept of uncertainty is essential to understanding finalized behavior. In fact, temporal specificity and event-behavior links (our own action effects) remain undefined until the event occurs. Thus, finalized behavior might be considered as a behavioral strategy for facing uncertainty. In new situations (e.g., starting a communicative exchange with a stranger), in which individuals exploit the majority of their cognitive resources, the degree of uncertainty is maximum.

Regarding motor preparation, defined as the action of an effector system on response production, different sub-processes are involved. It is therefore possible to define motor preparation as the set of operations that take place after a stimulus has been identified as significant but before the response is executed; that is, the selection of the appropriate answer to a specific input and the programming of a motor response output. In particular, it is assumed that, during the initial phases of context adaptation, cognitive structures influence each other through feed-forward processes aimed at the real-time regulation of resource allocation. By contrast, during the subsequent adaptation phases, when uncertainty and complexity factors are reduced, resource allocation is guided by automatic processes.

9.3.3 Self-monitoring and Meta-cognition

Monitoring and self-monitoring involve different cognitive functions, such as the ability to evaluate the outcomes of a communicative action, comparing them to initial hypotheses, and the ability to represent a situation by taking into account contextual variables. In particular, it is necessary for a subject to be able to represent his or her own competencies and those of the interlocutor. We refer to pragmatic implication but also to cognitive and meta-cognitive process interpretation. In the first case, *inferential abilities* are employed to evaluate the outcomes of one's actions with regard to predicted effects and actual outcome (*self-monitoring functions*); this competence is based on inferential processes regarding the cognitive, emotional, and behavioral effects of actions [1]. The second case draws on higher-order inferential processes related to the mental operations guiding our actions (*self-directed meta-cognition*) and the attribution of an epistemic state to other people (*hetero-directed meta-cognition*) (see [37]). Both competencies intersect with the whole communication process, since they are involved in the entire range of dynamics, from the initial phases of planning to interaction re-calibration.

Is there a common substrate of self-directed and hetero-directed meta-cognitive competencies? Recent studies evidenced the frontal lobes in meta-cognitive functions and specifically in the formulation of a theory of the mind. Moreover, there seems to be a direct relationship between specific deficits in the attentional system and in executive functions and the ability to formulate hypotheses about one's own mental contents and those of other people. Studies on individuals with lesions to prefrontal areas indicate a deficient representation of first- and second-level beliefs. Autistic individuals show a general inability to draw inferences relative to meta-cognitive states as well as compromised functioning of specific executive functions, such as strategies and goal-directed actions. It seems, therefore, that the two competencies share several properties, at least with regard to a common anatomico-functional substrate [38, 39].

9.4 The Contribution of Social Neuroscience to Communication

Only recently, social competencies have been considered as one of the pre-requisites for regulating the communicative exchange. The complex relation between meta-cognition and communication [40] includes empathy and emotional syntonization, as well as mentalization and the attribution of mental states. It is necessary to take into account the articulated ensemble of relational competencies that constitute the foundations of communicative mutual exchange. Competencies included in this field refer to specific dimensions such as: (1) the ability to infer one's own mental state and the mental states of other people (*mentalization functions*); (2) an understanding of *emotional states* as constitutive elements of communication and emotional syntonization ability; and (3) the ability to represent the *relational context* framing communicative interaction and to engage in communication *monitoring* and *self-monitoring* of communicative actions.

The new approach offered by *social neuroscience* directly investigates the relation between cortical and subcortical cerebral components and interactive processes. This perspective draws on a plurality of disciplines, such as the study of mentalization processes, emotional processes of self- and hetero-regulation, and conversation dynamics. For this reason, social neuroscience makes use of different and heterogeneous levels of analysis and a plurality of methodologies.

9.4.1 Models of the Mental States of Others

Essential to the communicative act is the ability to understand that others have beliefs, motivations, and thoughts. In this regard, research has considered especially two issues: (1) the definition of representational competencies aimed at the comprehension of other individuals as *intentional agents* [41, 42] and (2) *mentalization processes* characterizing one's own theory of mind and that of other people [43]. On a neurofunctional level, it is possible to distinguish a specific representation for individuals, as well as representations for other object categories [44]. In particular, the possibility to represent others, and their distinctive properties, as intentional agents is based on a specific semantic representation, defined through discrete categories that cannot overlap categories used for other objects [40].

Great attention has been given to the mentalization functions allowing representation of the other as an intentional agent and the attribution of consistency and invariance to some psychological features of other individuals (the other as a psychological entity). This last case refers to the fact that interlocutor representation is characterized by stable properties attributed to subjective identity, which allow individuals to predict the interlocutor's behavior and communicative choices. On the neuropsychological level, empirical evidence has identified specific correlates, related to the creation of stable impressions relative to the interlocutor's profile, localized in ample areas of the medial prefrontal cortex.

Of great interest is the specificity of these functions compared to a more general social competence. In this direction, neuropsychological research has examined the functional autonomy of socio-cognitive function in relation to other cognitive competencies (inference, hetero-attribution, etc.). In particular, it seems that the medial prefrontal cortex constitutes a common neural substrate for social cognition [45, 46, 47]; indeed, recent studies have evidenced distinct cortical areas specialized in the elaboration of information linked to the self (mental states, properties, actions, behaviors) [48] and in the elaboration of the mental states of other individuals. In

9

particular, the medial prefrontal cortex, right temporal junction, superior temporal sulcus, and fusiform gyrus appear to be involved in the elaboration of information concerning the mental states of other people. The medial prefrontal area appears to be active in the representation of mental states attributed to other human beings (and not to generic living beings).

9.4.2 Meta-cognition and Conversation Regulation

Meta-cognitive mechanisms have been investigated within the general domain of communicative interaction, in which mutual exchange dynamics are considered essential. Conversation can be represented as a finalized interaction among individuals within defined spatio-temporal coordinates and requiring specific meta-cognitive abilities (see previous paragraph).

The ensemble of mutually produced representations constitutes the cognitive background that ensures coherence and relevance to communicative dynamics: the representation of relevant information and the mutual exchange and sharing of knowledge shaping the common ground [49]. Recently, a branch of empirical research has focused on the basic elements of the communicative act, in terms of intentionalization and re-intentionalization processes. In addition, the concept of *mental model* has received great attention within the study of conversational pragmatics. According to this perspective, conversational and focal representational elements are progressively integrated into a speaker's mental models, increasing the set of shared reciprocal knowledge.

Those functions include interaction management and behavior regulation within social contexts. With regard to the ability to regulate one's own behavior as a function of conversational context requests, specific deficits in social communication competencies have been identified. Generally, those deficits have been classified as *interpersonal communication disorders* and include the inability to evaluate the coherence of inferred and represented contextual elements [50]. These deficits refer to the subject's inability to update or adapt his or her mental models to the real situation, and they are generally associated with deficits in wider competencies in the understanding of social contexts and in information contextualization. Gardner et al. [51] underlined that this inability to *contextualize events* and evaluate their *plausibility* accompanies the inability to understand the general meaning of conversational scripts. This task, typical of the right hemisphere, allows an individual to evaluate the probability or possibility that an event will happen. Patients with right hemisphere deficits cannot cope with incoherence and the violation of semantic plausibility of objects/events in specific situations. Finally, the impossibility of understanding the different levels of a speaker's *mutual knowledge* has been linked to deficits of a representational nature, typical of social cognition.

More analytically, paradigms concerned with conversation regulation show two relevant elements: *local coherence* and *global plausibility* in exchange regulation.

Coherence is based on the cohesion of the different parts of a discourse, on thematic progression (avoiding redundancy), logical coherence, and discourse pragmatic relevance [52].

A second fundamental element of conversational exchange is *turn-taking,* which concerns openings, closures, and turn management in relevant transactional contexts [53]. Speakers regulate their turns, selecting themselves (e.g., by increasing their tone of voice) or their interlocutor (e.g., by asking a question). An interesting case is that of paired-turns, i.e., adjacent components that depend on one another, such as initial greetings and offering/refusal. The type of sentence produced by the speaker and the influence of contextual variables are further relevant aspects of conversation, since they impact directly on interpretative processes. For instance, the direct/indirect nature of requests, determined by speaker's communicative intentions, directly affects the listener's ability to correctly decode the speaker's intention (re-intentionalization).

References

1. Green GM (1996) Pragmatics and natural language understanding. Erlbaum, Hillsdale, New Jersey
2. Sperber D, Wilson D (1986) Relevance: communication and cognition. Oxford University Press, Oxford
3. Balconi M (2008) Neuropragmatica [Neuropragmatics]. Aracne, Roma
4. Marraffa M, Meini C (2005) La mente sociale: le basi cognitive della comunicazione [The social mind: cognitive bases of communication]. Laterza, Roma
5. Csibra G (2004) Teleological and referential understanding of action in infancy. In: Frith CD, Wolpert DM (eds) The neuroscience of social interaction: decoding, imitating and influencing the actions of others. Oxford University Press, Oxford, pp 23-44
6. Tomasello M (1999) The cultural origins of human cognition. Harvard University Press, Cambridge, MA
7. Balconi M (2002) Neuropsicologia della comunicazione. In: Anolli L (ed) Psicologia della comunicazione. Il Mulino, Bologna
8. Frith U, Frith CD (2004) Development and neurophysiology of mentalizing. In: Frith CD, Wolpert DM (eds) The neuroscience of social interaction: decoding, imitating and influencing the actions of others. Oxford University Press, Oxford, pp 45-75
9. Gallese V (2004) The manifold nature of interpersonal relations: the quest for a common mechanism. In: Frith CD, Wolpert DM (2004) The neuroscience of social interaction: decoding, imitating and influencing the actions of others. Oxford University Press, Oxford, pp 159-182
10. Dennett D (2001) Are we explaining consciousness yet? Cognition 79:221-237
11. Zelazo PD (1999) Language, levels of consciousness, and the development of intentional action. In: Zelazo PD, Astington JW, Olson DR (eds) Developing theories of intention: social understanding and self control. Erlbaum, Hillsdale, New Jersey, pp 95-118
12. Balconi M (2006) Psicologia degli stati di coscienza: dalla coscienza percettiva alla consapevolezza di sé [Psychology of consciousness: from perceptual consciousness to self awareness]. LED, Milano
13. Kinsbourne M (1996) What qualifies a representation for a role in consciousness? In: Cohen JD, Schooler JW (eds) Scientific approaches to consciousness: the twenty-fifth annual Carnegie symposium on cognition. Erlbaum, Hillsdale, New Jersey

9

14. Spence DP, Smith GW (1977) Experimenter bias against subliminal perception? Comments on a replication. Brit J Psychol 68:279-280
15. Kinsbourne M (1988) Integrated field theory of consciousness. In: Marcel AE, Bisiach E (eds) Consciousness in contemporary science. Clarendon Press, Oxford, pp 239-256
16. Gazzaniga MS (1998) The mind's past. University of California Press, Berkeley
17. Baars BJ (2003) How does a serial, integrated, and very limited stream of consciousness emerge from a nervous system that is mostly unconscious, distributed, parallel, and of enormous capacity? In: Baars BJ, Banks WP, Newman JB (eds) Essential sources in the scientific study of consciousness. The MIT Press, Cambridge, Massachusetts, pp 1123-1130
18. Gazzaniga MS (1996) The cognitive neuroscience. The MIT Press, Cambridge, MA
19. Povinelli DJ, Bering JM (2002) The mentality of apes revisited. Curr Dir Psychol Sci 11:115-119
20. Balconi M, Mazza G (2009) Consciousness and emotion: ERP modulation and attentive vs. pre-attentive elaboration of emotional facial expressions by backward masking. Mot Emot 33:113-124
21. Balconi M, Crivelli D (2009) FRN and P300 ERP effect modulation in response to feedback sensitivity: the contribution of punishment-reward system (BIS/BAS) and behaviour identification of action. Neurosci Res 66:162-172
22. Shallice T (1988) From neuropsychology to mental structure. Cambridge University Press, Cambridge
23. Bottini G, Paulesu E, Sterzi R et al (1995) Modulation of conscious experience in peripheral sensory stimuli. Nature 376:778-780
24. Feyereisen P (1988) Non verbal communication. In: Rose FC, Whurr R, Wyke MA (eds) Aphasia. Whurr, London, pp 46-81
25. Baddeley A (1996) Exploring the central executive. Q J Exp Psychol-A 49:5-28
26. Gazzaniga MS (1997) Conversations in the cognitive neurosciences. The MIT Press, Cambridge, MA
27. Vallar G, Baddeley AD (1987) Phonological short-term store and sentence processing. Cogn Neuropsychol 4:417-438
28. Vallar G, Baddeley AD (1984) Fractionation of working memory: neuropsychological evidence for a phonological short-term store. J Verbl Learn Verb Be 23:151-161
29. Belleville S, Peretz I, Arguin H (1992) Contribution of articulatory reharsal to short-term memory: evidence from a selective disruption. Brain Lang 43:713-746
30. Martin RC, Feher E (1990) The consequences of reduced memory span for the comprehension of semantic versus syntactic information. Brain Lang 38:1-20
31. McCarthy RA, Warrington EK (1990) Cognitive neuropsychology: a clinical introduction. Academic Press, San Diego
32. Waters GS, Caplan D, Hildebrandt N (1991) On the structure of verbal short-term memory and its functional role in sentence comprehension: evidence from neuropsychology. Cogn Neuropsychol 8:82-126
33. Martin RC (1993) Short-term memory and sentence processing: evidence from neuropsychology. Mem Cognition 21:176-183
34. Damasio AR (2000) The feeling of what happens: body and emotion in the making of consciousness. Vintage, London
35. Sommerhoff G (2000) Understanding consciousness. Its function and brain processes. Sage, London
36. Stuss DT, Alexander MP, Benson DF (1997) Frontal lobe functions. In: Trimble MR, Cummings JL (eds) Contemporary behavioral neurology. Butterworth-Heineman, Boston, pp 169-187
37. Frith CD, Wolpert DM (2004) The neuroscience of social interaction: decoding, imitating and influencing the actions of others. Oxford University Press, New York

38. Baron-Cohen S (1995) Mindblindness: an essay on autism and theory of mind. The MIT Press, Cambridge, MA
39. Frith CD (2003) Neural hermeneutics: how brains interpret minds. Keynote lecture, 9th Annual Meeting of the Organization of Human Brain Mapping, New York
40. Mitchell JP, Mason MF, Macrae CN, Banaji MR (2006) Thinking about others: the neural substrates of social cognition. In: Cacioppo JT, Visser PS, Pickett CL (eds) Social neuroscience: people thinking other people. MIT Press, Cambridge, pp 63-82
41. Morris JS, Frith CD, Perret DI et al (1996) A differential neural response in the human amygdale to fearful and happy facial expressions. Nature 383:812-815
42. Philips ML, Young AW, Senior C et al (1997) A specific neural substrates for perceiving facial expressions of disgust. Nature 389:495-498
43. Frith CD (2007) Making up the mind: how the brain creates our mental world. Blackwell Publishing, Oxford
44. Caramazza A, Shelton JR (1998) Domain-specific knowledge systems in the brain: the animate-inanimate distinction. J Cognitive Neurosci 10:1-34
45. Adolphs R (2003) Cognitive neuroscience of human social behaviour. Nat Rev Neurosci 4:165-178
46. Crivelli D, Balconi M (2009) Trends in social neuroscience: from biological motion to joint action. Neuropsychol Trends 6:71-93
47. Gallagher HL, Frith CD (2003) Functional imaging of "theory of mind". Trends Cogn Sci 7:77-83
48. Blackemore SJ, Decety J (2001) From the perception of action to the understanding of intention. Nat Neurosci 10:561-567
49. Sperber D, Wilson D (2003) Pragmatics, modularity and mind reading. Mind Lang 17:3-23
50. Kaplan JA, Brownell HH, Jacobs JR, Gardner H (1990) The effects of right hemisphere damage on the pragmatic interpretation of conversational remarks. Brain Lang 38:315-333
51. Gardner H, Brownell HH, Wapner W, Michelow D (1983) Missing the point: the role of the right hemisphere in the processing of complex linguistic material. In: Perecman E (ed) Cognitive processing in the right hemisphere. Academic Press, New York, pp 169-182
52. Charolles M (1986) Grammaire de texte, théorie du discour, narrativité. Pratiques 11-12:133-154
53. Schegloff EA (1972) Sequencing in conversational openings. In: Gumperz JJ, Hymes DH (eds) Directions in sociolinguistics. Holt, New York, pp 346-380

The Neuropsychology of Nonverbal Communication: The Facial Expressions of Emotions

10

M. Balconi

10.1 Introduction

The facial expressions of emotion probably do not exclusively serve an emotional purpose, but instead can be related to different functions. In fact, a broad domain of information can be conveyed through facial displays. In our interactions with others, facial expressions enable us to communicate effectively, and they work in conjunction with spoken words as well as other, nonverbal acts. Among the expressive elements that contribute to the communication of emotion, facial expressions are considered as *communicative signals* [1]. In fact, facial expressions are central features of the social behavior of most nonhuman primates and they are powerful stimuli in human communication. Moreover, faces are crucial channels of *social cognition*, because of their high interpersonal value, and they permit the intentions of others to be deciphered. Thus, facial recognition may indirectly reflect the encoding and storage of *social acts*.

Recent research has shown that the perception of expression is much more complex than the simple labeling of an individual's behavior. Those studies of facial expression stressed the developmental pathway of emotions, to what extent the information they convey is captured by discrete categories or scalar dimensions, whether emotions have distinct biological correlates, etc. For example, according to dimensional theorists, valence and arousal organize the connections between facial expression and emotions. However, even if one rejects a specific one-to-one correspondence between facial expression and cortical sites, certain specific dimensions appear to be critical in activating cerebral mechanisms, such as the arousal and valence of the emotional stimulus. From the neuropsychological point of view, an

M. Balconi (✉)
Department of Psychology, Catholic University of Milan, Milan, Italy

analysis of the neural control of facial expression provides a window into at least some aspects of the neural system involved in emotion.

10.2 Facial Expressions: Discrete Categories or Dimensions?

A central question in the field of emotional facial comprehension is whether emotions are better represented as discrete systems [2, 3] or as interrelated entities that differ along global dimensions, such as valence, activity, etc. [4]. From the *categorical perspective*, it is possible to identify discrete emotions, and it is reasonable to propose that the universal component in the facial expression of emotions is the connection between particular facial configurations and specific emotions. By contrast, in the *dimensional approach* emotions are not discrete but better conceptualized as differing in the degree of one or another dimension. As Ellsworth [5] has argued, the existence of distinct facial expressions supports major evidence for holistic emotion programs that cannot be broken down into smaller units. Discrete models assume that the facial expressions of some basic emotions are innate, based on evidence of discrete emotional expressions in infants. Moreover, there is considerable agreement indicating distinct, prototypical facial signals that, across a variety of cultures, can be reliably recognized as corresponding to at least six different emotions (happiness, sadness, surprise, disgust, anger, and fear). The fact that these expressions are widely recognized suggests that meaningful information is encoded in them.

An alternative view is that of Izard [6, 7], who elaborated the *differential emotions theory*. This integrative model shares some of the main tenets of the discrete perspective. Referring to Darwin's hypothesis and considering cross-cultural data as well as ethological research on nonhuman facial displays, the author proposed that the facial expressions of a few basic emotions are innate and that it is possible to identify examples of discrete emotional expressions in young infants, since in this group there is some evidence of the early emergence and morphological stability of certain facial patterns. Nevertheless, Izard discussed universality and distinguished it from the problem of innateness, but while universality is generally supported, innateness has been more difficult to examine. In parallel, even though universal prototypical patterns have been found for different emotions, these findings have not enabled researchers to interpret facial expressions as unambiguous indicators of emotions in spontaneous interactions. More specifically, it is unclear whether certain facial expressions express emotions; that is, while it was assumed that these expressions are caused by emotion, it is necessary to establish whether there are intrinsic links between facial expression and emotion per se.

In the above-mentioned *dimensional perspective*, facial expressions are not signals of specific emotions; instead, a decoder either detects or infers information about what the displayer is doing, the displayer's attentiveness, his/her pleasantness, and the degree of arousal [4, 8-11]. A main topic in this approach is the cognitive significance of facial comprehension, i.e., the role of the decoder's evaluation processing in attributing a meaning to a particular facial expression. Specifically, pleasantness and arousal are construed as two orthogonal dimensions of a psychological judgment space within which emotion labels can be represented. In this regard, several researchers have analyzed facial expressions as indicators of *appraisal processes*. Smith and Scott [12], for example, proposed four dimensions of meaning, organized by adaptive functions, into which facial components cluster: (1) *pleasantness* of the emotional state, (2) the *attentional activity* associated with the emotional state, (3) *arousal*, and (4) *personal agency* and control. The hedonistic dimension is associated with the perception of goal obstacles and anticipated effort. The attentional component reflects the novelty of the situation and the degree of certainty about the circumstances. Emotional experiences would be expected to cluster in the dimensionally structured space, thereby creating families of emotion, with each family containing overlapping sets of components.

How we can characterize which emotion is expressed? The information contained in facial expressions is that which is common in raising appraisal expectations, evoking affect and behavior expectations in interactions. It is what is common to the various conditions under which a given expression arises and to the various emotional and nonemotional states that may elicit a given expression. Facial expression represents the manner in which the individual at that particular moment relates to the environment [13]. It is the position taken: acceptance or refusal and thus activity or lack thereof. Fridlund [14] called facial expressions *states of action readiness*, i.e., states of readiness to establish, maintain, or change a particular kind of relationship with some object in the environment. The emotion-expression relationship is greatly clarified by the componential approach to emotions: emotions are structures made up of moderately correlated components, including affect, appraisal, action disposition, and physiological responses. Thus, we can conceptualize facial expression as an *expressive behavior*, carrying expressive information as: (1) a vehicle of *intention attribution* and comprehension; (2) *relational activity* proper, i.e., behavior that modifies the individual's relationship to the environment; (3) *social signals* to orient the behavior of others, thus serving as nonverbal requests or commands; and (4) *activation* (defined as tonic readiness to act) and *deactivation manifestations*.

10.2.1 What About Intention Attribution?

Now we can ask explicitly whether the meaning of a facial expression depends on the context in which it occurs. Common sense suggests that the answer is yes, even if most research on facial expressions presupposes that they have meaning independent of their context and that context plays no essential role in the recognition of emotions from facial expressions. Expressions are embedded in a context, occurring in a particular time and place, such that we have to assume a *figure-ground interaction* between facial expressions and context. In fact, the meaning of a facial display to a decoder is a function of how the facial feature is related to other features of the displayer and the displayer's context, but also to the decoder's context. Facial expressions occur in context and are detected and interpreted in context. Emotional meaning may then be attributed by the decoder to the displayer, since the perception of emotion is more an *act of attribution* that comes towards the end of a sequence and is a contingent act rather than a necessary or automatic one.

Several empirical studies have shown that predictable facial expressions occur in emotion-eliciting interpersonal situations. Thus, some models have focused on the social and ethological valence of facial expressions, as well as on the social interaction significance of facial displays. The ability to recognize facial expressions is important for effective social interaction and for gathering information about the environment.

The reciprocal relationship between encoder and decoder in emotional attribution evokes a second representational problem in face comprehension: the role of the *intention attribution*. The face is more than a means for communicating emotions. It is also a vehicle for communicating intentions to conspecifics, since inferring the intentions of others is a natural ability that we employ in everyday situations. For example, eye gaze and the processing of facial and other biologically relevant movements all contribute to the evaluation of intent in others [15]. Eye contact is particularly meaningful in non-human and human primates. Monkeys communicate threat and submission through facial displays as part of a complex facial system. In the same manner, facial movements are important for recognizing facial expressions and for attributing intentions and goals to others. That is, facial expression in everyday life are not static but are constructed by movements of the eyes, mouth, and other facial elements.

Before one is able to distinguish and recognize different facial expressions, one must use facial expressions to read emotional states in others. For example, by 12–14 months of age, infants can use adults' facial expressions as referents or indicators of objects in the environment, avoiding objects towards which adults display negative facial reactions, such as disgust. In addition, the evolution of pleasure/approach and disgust/avoidance reactions to food has been important for survival and may have evolved in parallel with the ability to recognize facial expressions in a context of non-verbal social communication, thus serving both the producer and the decoder [16].

10.2.2 Facial Expressions as Social Signals

Facial expression production and perception are inherent and rule-governed processes, and the ability to perceive and discriminate among intentions from facial expressions clearly involves an information-processing system. Ability in facial expression identification and in other prosocial behaviors forms a cluster of related abilities that may be associated with evolutionary fitness. Social influences on the production and interpretation of facial expression are also important to consider, since the species-specific topographies of facial displays are modified by cultural and environmental influences. For example, neonatal responses are modified during the first year of life, possibly as a result of reinforcement within a cultural context. Caregivers encourage or discourage infants' emotional responses depending on cultural norms, and there are associated observable emotional displays or lack of displays in these infants.

But, how do we attribute emotional intention to others based on facial expression? Goldman's model proposed a neuropsychological explanation. This approach holds that people typically execute mind-reading by a simulation process in attributing an emotion to a face. The decoder arrives at a mental attribution by simulating, replicating, or reproducing in his or her own mind the state of another person [17]. According to simulation theory, these results are explainable by the core idea that the decoder selects a mental state for attribution after reproducing or enacting within himself the very state in question, that is, attempting to replicate the other's mental state by undergoing the same or similar mental process as the one in question. Of course, this account assumes that there is enough information in the facial expression itself to uniquely select an appropriate corresponding emotional state. Simulation theory proposes that a decoder selects an emotional category to assign to a person by producing that emotion himself, and then seeing which emotion has an appropriate link to the observed facial expression.

Based on a *heuristic procedure* (generate-and-test), the decoder starts by hypothesizing a certain emotion as the possible cause of the displayed face and proceeds to enact that emotion, that is, to produce a facsimile of it in his own system. The course of facsimile construction includes the production of the corresponding natural facial expression, or at least a neural instruction to the facial musculature to construct the relevant expression. If the resulting facial expression matches the expression observed in the target, then the hypothesized emotion is confirmed and the decoder imputes that emotion to the target. If a person is impaired in the relevant emotional area and cannot enact that emotion or produce a facsimile thereof, he or she cannot generate the relevant face-related downstream activity necessary to recognize the emotion.

10.2.3 Facial Expressions of Emotion as Cognitive Functions

The face conveys a variety of information about individuals. Some of this information is visually derived and therefore can be accessed solely on the basis of the physical attributes of the physiognomy irrespective of the identity of the individual (gender, age, etc.), whereas other information is semantically derived. In the latter case, it can be accessed only after the perceived representation of the face makes contact with the corresponding stored representation, from which biographical information about the individual can then be reactivated. Inquiry into the processes underlying the perception and recognition of faces has led to the development of models that describe the various types of physical facial information so as to achieve as veridical a description as possible of the attributes and properties of a perceived face. This kind of description serves as the basis on which all face-related processes begin. Subsequently, different combinations of facial features convey pertinent information about gender, age, or expression, such that different operations must be performed to access the different bits of information contained in a facial description.

Firstly, the dissociation among different stages of face processing has been well documented and together with behavioral observation and experimental evidence has led to the development of the well-known cognitive model of face recognition proposed by Bruce and Young [18]. This model of facial recognition is expressed in terms of processing pathways and modules for facial recognition. In fact, from the face, people derive different types of information, which the authors called *codes*. These codes are not themselves the functional components of the face processing system; rather, they are the products of the operation of the functional components. Specifically, seven types of codes can be derived from faces: *pictorial*, *structural*, *visually derived semantics*, *identity-specific semantics*, *name*, *expression*, and *facial speech* (movements of the lips). Figure 10.1 shows Bruce and Young's functional model.

In one's relation to others, the pictorial code provides information about lighting and grain, in other words, the pictorial code corresponds to the 2D image of the face. By contrast, the structural code captures the aspect of the configuration of a face that distinguishes it from other faces. In considering pictorial and structural codes, the former is a description of a picture and should not be equated with view-specific derived information. Nevertheless a pictorial code cannot by itself accomplish the task of facial recognition despite changes in head angle, expression, age, etc. From a picture of a face, another, more abstract, visual representation must be established that can mediate recognition. Accordingly, we proceed to derive structural codes for faces that capture those aspects of a face's structure essential to distinguish that face from other faces. It is the more abstract structural code that mediates the everyday recognition of familiar faces, and some areas of the face provide more information about a person's identity than others.

10.2.4
The Stage Processing Model

While the evidence favors functional components in the processing of human faces, we still need to examine how the information derived from the face is used. As Bruce and Young proposed, the different types of information may be viewed as functional "codes" such that to a certain extent facial recognition can be described in terms of the sequential access of different codes (Fig. 10.1).

The main issues related to the conceptualization of codes can be synthesized in two questions: (1) What are the different information codes used in facial processing? (2) What functional components are responsible for the generation and access of these different codes? Firstly, there is a distinction to be drawn between the products of a process and the processes themselves. In substance, we have to consider some of the procedures that generate and access the codes we have described, thereby focusing on the relationships between a number of broad functional components. A function of the cognitive system underlying this structure is to direct attention to the usable components in a specific context. Thus, as well as passively recognizing expressions, identities, etc., from a face, we also encode certain kinds of information selectively and strategically.

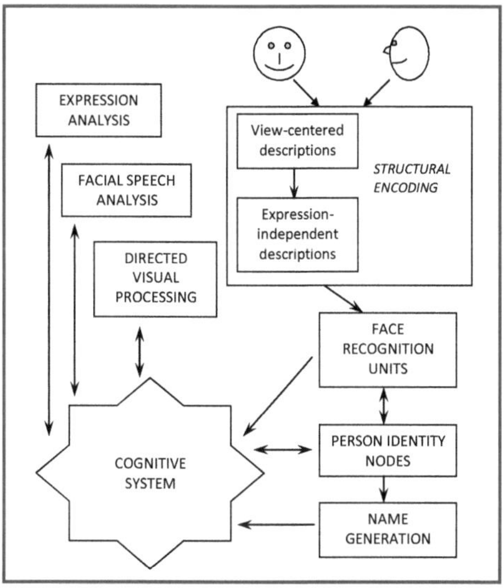

Fig. 10.1 Bruce and Young model of face recognition [18]

Codes differ in terms of the cognitive and functional sub-processes they represent. Indeed several models of facial recognition incorporate an initial structural encoding mechanism with physiognomic features as input and an integrated representation of face as output. The resulting structural code allows the identification of particular exemplars of faces despite changes in viewing angle, expression, lighting, age, etc. According to such models, facial identification is achieved by the combined operation of facial recognition units and semantic nodes. The facial recognition units select the pre-stored face model that best fits the currently structured perceptual representation, and the semantic nodes make available the entire knowledge associated in semantic memory regarding the particular facial model selected. The domain specificity of the structural encoder and its categorized output representation prevent facial recognition from attempting to match the resulting representation to all possible object models. Indeed, in the absence of such specificity, facial recognition is inhibited and becomes inefficient.

A functional dissociation was described between a specific visual mechanism responsible for *structural encoding* and a higher-level mechanism responsible for associating the structural representations of a face with *semantic information*, such as expression or identity [11, 19]. Thus, it has become clear that we are not only able to derive information concerning the person's likely age, sex, etc., but that we also can interpret the meaning of that person's facial expression, and we refer to this as the formation of an expression code. The most striking support for different systems for processing facial identity and facial emotions comes from a double dissociation between the recognition of people and the identification of emotion, such as occurs in prosopagnosic disturbances. Paragraph 10.2.5 describes the empirical support in favor of the dissociation between different types of codes, as well as their functional significance.

Research into the rules governing facial recognition has focused mainly on the role of structural encoding in facial identification. For example, these studies have examined how variations in viewing conditions influence facial recognition or stimulus configuration. Some of the experiments in facial processing were not explicitly designed to investigate differences in the processing of facial identity and facial expressions, but instead examined the effects of changes in appearance. The empirical results suggested that a single view of a face may contain enough invariant information to allow subsequent recognition despite moderate changes in pose and expressions.

Neuropsychological and cognitive research have jointly made evident the intrinsic distinction between the face and other perceptual stimuli. The contribution of cognitive neuroscience has been to identify the neural substrates involved in extracting the different types of information conveyed by faces. Each of these neural substrates is a face-specific processing component and together they form a face-specific system. Moreover, the main result of cognitive neuroscience with respect to facial processing is the possibility to characterize the *functional organization* of the facial processing system. In particular, it has allowed illustration of the components of that system, a description of what each component does and how it works, as well as an understanding of how the components interact in facial processing tasks.

An important direction for empirical research is to determine more precisely the role of each of the functional components implicated in facial processing, such as structural, semantic, and expression codes. These efforts will require both cognitive and neuropsychological approaches. In addition, there are increasing sources of data showing that the recognition of specific emotions depends on the existence of partially distinct systems. Currently, there is much debate as to whether a distributed neural model of facial perception requires a more exhaustive perspective. For example, the distinction between different types of emotions (such as positive and negative emotions) could be a heuristic factor that conditions the neural correlates underlying facial decoding. Similarly, analysis of the difference between stimuli of high- and low-level arousal may be of interest in comprehending the brain's mechanism of facial decoding.

Finally, an important issue in the neuropsychology of facial comprehension is related to the contributions of the left and right hemispheres. Distinct cortical functions were initially related to the two hemispheres, that is right and left lateralization effects were found. Emotion recognition by facial expression was originally differentiated from emotion production. But as yet, there is no clear resolution as to which model best fits all the experimental literature, since more than one variable has shown to be effective in facial expression lateralization, such as the type of emotion implicated (positive/negative), the function of that emotion (approach/withdrawal), the processing stage (encoding or decoding), as well as the type of task (emotion recognition or other tasks). Thus, it is now obvious that the search for a single, bipolar principle encompassing the functional properties of the two hemispheres is futile. Nevertheless, following a description of both the functional neuroanatomy of the approach and withdrawal systems, differences in brain activation were found and their relation to affective style was described. Moreover, individual differences in brain lateralization have been revealed by different neuropsychological measures.

10.2.5 Structural and Semantic Mechanisms of Emotional Facial Processing. Empirical Evidence

An increasing amount of research has analyzed the cognitive and neuropsychological features of facial comprehension [20]. Specifically, positron emission tomography (PET) studies [21, 22], functional magnetic resonance imaging (fMRI) [23-25], and event-related potentials (ERPs) [26, 27] have underlined the brain's specificity in encoding emotions.

Relevant evidence supporting the functional specificity of brain mechanisms responsible for facial processing is provided by psychophysiological studies addressing ERPs of long latencies [28, 29]. Different face-specific ERP components are likely to reflect successive stages in the processing of faces–from the perceptual analysis and structural encoding of facial components to the classification and identification of individual facial stimuli. To understand whether and how such ERP components are related to face-specific processing stages, it is essential to study how these stages are influenced by experimental manipulations known to have an impact on the quality of facial perception and recognition. In particular, studies using ERP measures have identified neural correlates in which those for facial detection are larger than those for many other stimuli, including houses, cars, or eyes [30, 31].

The structural encoding process is probably the final stage in visual analysis and its product is an abstract sensory representation of a face, i.e., a representation that is independent of context or viewpoint. Likewise, procedures that disrupt facial patterns in terms of their perceptual details should influence the comprehension of facial stimuli, as shown by an increasing N170 peak amplitude [32]. In addition, several experimental manipulations have been aimed at understanding how the structural face-decoding mechanism functions. Isolated eyes or a combination of inner components presented without the face contour elicited an N170 that was significantly larger than that elicited by a full face.

Additionally, a functional dissociation was revealed between a specific visual mechanism responsible for the structural encoding of faces and a higher-level mechanism responsible for associating the structural representation of a face with semantic information, such as emotional expression [33, 34]. ERP modulations sensitive to face semantic encoding have been observed at longer latencies. In a study in which ERPs were recorded in response to familiar faces as well as to unfamiliar faces and to houses, unfamiliar faces elicited an enhanced negativity between 250 ms and 550 ms (called the N400 effect), which was followed by an enhanced positivity beyond 500 ms post-stimulus (P600). These effects were maximal for the first presentation of individual familiar faces and were attenuated for subsequent presentations of the same faces. Because of their sensitivity to face familiarity, the N400 and P600 effects are likely to indicate processes involved in the recognition and identification of faces. Specifically, N400 and P600 reflect brain mechanisms involved in the activation of stored representations of faces and subsequent activations of semantic memory, while the N170 could be linked to the pre-categorical perceptual analysis of faces. In fact, an N400-like effect has been observed for non-familiar *vs* familiar faces [29, 30], unknown *vs* known faces, matching *vs* non-matching tasks, non-semantic *vs* semantic matching tasks, and face-feature matching tasks. For example, N400 was reported to be larger for non-matching words and for faces [35].

To summarize, the N400 effect, initially detected during semantically incongruent sentence ending in language [36, 37], has offered important insights into the organization of semantic memory. It is considered to reflect information processing not only in the linguistic domain, but also in the accessing of semantic representational systems [38]. It therefore has been proposed that N400 is modulated not only by semantically incongruous words, but also when a stimulus activates any representational system in memory. N400 was considered to reflect access to and activity within the semantic memory system, and it may show additional neural response to semantically incongruous information of complex stimuli.

An analogous paradigm has been used in several recent ERP studies of facial processing [39]. The general findings were that, relative to congruent or matching faces, incongruent or mismatching faces elicit an N400 response, as described above. Moreover, Münte et al. [40] reported an interesting result: ERP differences between congruent and incongruent faces had different scalp topographies for identity and expression tasks. This finding was interpreted as indicating that different neural substrates subserve identity and expression analysis.

Based on these empirical results, we can delineate neurophysiological correlates of the processing of faces, those for identity and those for expression, thus supporting cognitive models of facial processing. In fact, large differences have been found in the timing and spatial features of ERPs for the two different face-processing functions. The ERP effect appears to qualify as the physiological counterpart of the proposed modularity of facial processing. The earliest differences in identity matching were found at about 200 ms, whereas the earliest effects in expression matching were apparent only at 450 ms (Fig 10.2). This time difference suggests that structure processing required for the recognition of a person follows two different time-courses, with expression matching occurring considerably later in time.

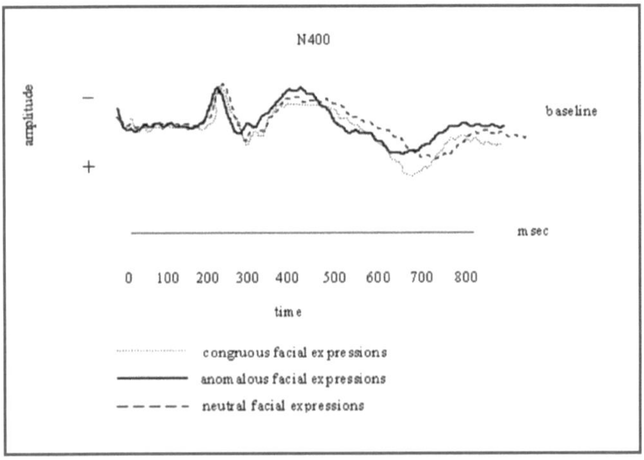

Fig. 10.2 Grand-average ERPs elicited by congruous, anomalous, and neutral facial expressions (10 electrodes)

10.3
Neuropsychological Correlates of Emotional Facial Processing

Is there evidence of specific brain, i.e., cortical and subcortical, correlates of facial processing? Recently, an explicative model of cortical network implicated in face processing was described [21]. This distributed human neural system for facial perception is diagrammed in Figure 10.3. According to the model, two important components are assumed to be processed in the face: invariant facial representation and changeable facial aspects, such as facial expression, eye gaze, and lip movements. The model is hierarchical and is divided into a core system and an extended system. The core system is composed of three bilateral regions in the occipitotemporal visual extrastriate cortex and includes the inferior occipital gyri, the lateral fusiform gyrus, and the superior temporal sulcus. Haxby [21] used PET to examine areas of activation in response to the encoding and recognition of faces. The respective activation patterns showed dissociation between the neural systems involved in these two processes. Facial recognition, compared with the encoding task, activated the right prefrontal cortex, anterior cingulated cortex, bilateral inferior parietal cortex, and the cerebellum. Specifically, the right prefrontal cortex was activated only during the recognition task and not during the encoding task.

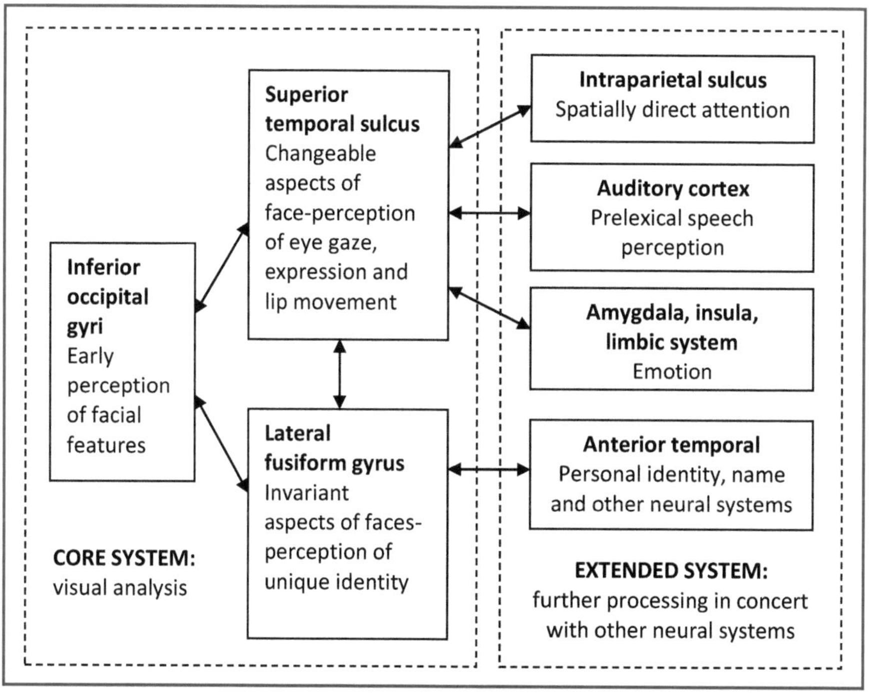

Fig. 10.3 The different neural correlates of facial comprehension

10.3.1 Regional Brain Support for Face-specific-processing?

In humans, facial expressions and identity processing, in spite of activating separate pathways, use similar processing mechanisms. The processing of facial expressions activates specific brain regions responsible for emotion processing. For example, the amygdala is responsible for fear processing [41], and the insula for processing disgust [42]. Facial processing occurs within the fusiform gyrus [43]. The mechanism and location of facial expression perception, including configural and categorical processing (see Chapter 1), are still widely debated. In a recent publication, Kanwisher and colleagues [23] examined the role of the fusiform gyrus in facial perception. This area can be viewed as a specialized module for facial perception and was accordingly termed the *fusiform face area* (FFA) (Fig. 10.4). Experiments revealed that the FFA responded more strongly to the viewing of intact rather than scrambled faces, and to frontal views of faces rather than frontal views of houses. FFA activation seems also to be dependent on the level of attention paid to facial stimuli: when facial stimuli appear outside the focus of attention, activity is reduced. These observations support the involvement of the FFA in facial perception (Fig. 10.2).

Taking into account clinical findings, impaired facial processing has been observed in a group of subjects with autism spectrum disorders (ASD). Deficits in social cognition, which include inactivity in response to the faces of others and failure to make appropriate eye contact, suggest that individuals with ADS have not developed typical facial expertise, generally relying on feature-based analysis of the face rather than configural processing. In an experiment of Schultz et al. [44], the autistic group showed significantly more activation in the right inferior temporal gyrus than in the right fusiform gyrus. According to the authors, the laterality differences support the claim that facial processing in autistic individuals proceeds by an object-based processing strategy, which activates the inferior temporal gyrus [45].

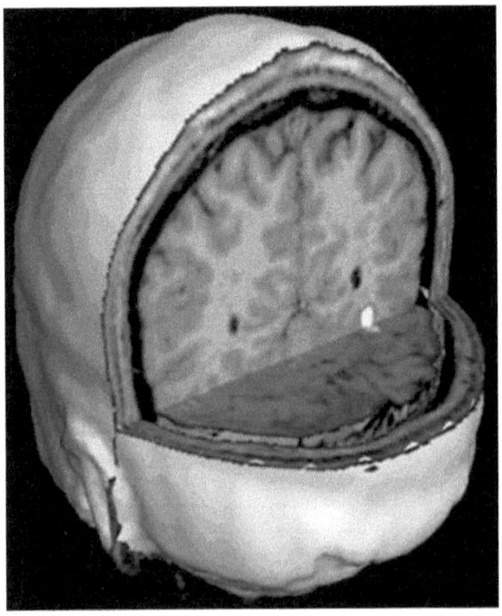

Fig. 10.4 Representation of the fusiform face area (FFA)

Deficits in the processing of facial expressions are obviously part of the pattern of impaired social skills of ASD individuals, but the deficits can also involve how autistic individuals process facial expressions [24].

10.3.2
The Role of the Frontal and Temporal Lobes and of the Limbic Circuit in Emotion Decoding

10.3.2.1
The Frontal Lobe

Support for the *orbitofrontal cortex* as a major area for generalized emotional facial processing comes from two sources of evidence. First, patient research has found that orbitofrontal damage is associated with impairments in identifying emotional expressions. Second, a PET study found that the orbitofrontal cortex is activated in response to emotional rather than neutral faces [46].

The frontal lobe is a vast area, representing 30% of the neocortex, and it is made up of several functionally distinct regions nonetheless synthesizable into three categories: motor, premotor, and prefrontal. The motor cortex is responsible for movements of the distal musculature, such as the fingers. The premotor cortex selects the movements to be made. The prefrontal cortex controls the cognitive processes so that the appropriate movements are selected at the correct place and time. This latter selection may be controlled by internalized information, or it may be made in response to context. The prefrontal cortex can be further subdivided with respect to response selection related to internal versus external information: the dorsolateral region and the inferior frontal region. The dorsolateral cortex is hypothesized to have evolved for the selection of behavior based on temporal memory, which is a form of internalized knowledge. Individuals whose temporal memory is defective become dependent on environmental cues to determine their behavior. The inferior frontal region is hypothesized to have a role in the control of response selection in context. Social behavior in particular is context dependent. People with inferior frontal lesions have context difficulties in social situations. During emotional tasks, and especially with facial emotion encoding and decoding, the spontaneous facial expressions of frontal lobe patients are reduced, in contrast to their ability for spontaneous talking. In addition, subjects with frontal lobe deficits (both right and left) are impaired in matching photographs showing fear and disgust [47].

10.3.2.2
The Temporal Lobe

Another important area implicated in facial processing is the temporal lobe, which includes neocortical tissue as well as the limbic cortex and subcortical structures (amygdala, hippocampus). The temporal cortex is rich in connections from sensory systems, especially visual and auditory systems, and in connections to and from the frontal lobe. In addition, it has major connections with the amygdala, which is presumed to play a central role in emotional behavior. One obvious difference between the left and right temporal cortices is that the left is involved in language processing, whereas the right is involved in facial processing. In the production of facial expression, some studies have found that subjects with temporal lobe lesions produce as many spontaneous expressions as seen in normal subjects. In the recognition of facial expression, the ability of subjects with left temporal lobe lesions to match the six basic facial expressions to photographs of spontaneous facial expressions was the same as that of normal subjects [48, 49].

10.3.2.3 The Limbic Contribution

In considering the limbic mechanisms that may be important in the differential hemispheric emotional characteristics, we can stress the interaction of lateralization with the functional differentiation between dorsal and ventral cortical pathways. It was proposed that right hemisphere specialization for the spatial functions of the dorsal cortical pathway may be relevant to both the attentional and the emotional deficits observed following right hemisphere damage. The right hemisphere may be responsible for emotional surveillance so that when this capacity is diminished following a lesion the patient fails to recognize the significance of emotionally important information. In this view, denial and indifference represent a kind of emotional neglect. Other authors have suggested that the left hemisphere's affective characteristics may have evolved in line with its elaboration of the motivational and cognitive functions of the ventral limbic circuitry. Although it is difficult to investigate, the relation between limbic and cortical systems seems to hold important clues to cognitive-affective interactions at the personality level.

10.3.2.4 The Contribution of the Amygdala

Theorists who support a model of discrete emotional expressions argue that the perception of different facial expressions involves distinct regions of the central nervous system. Specifically, it was shown that the perception of a fearful face activates regions in the left amygdala. In addition, lesion studies indicate that the perception of different emotions is associated with different brain regions. Bilateral lesions to the amygdala impair the ability to recognize fearful facial expression and localization but not the ability to recognize facial expressions of sadness, disgust, or happiness.

The amygdala is well-placed anatomically to integrate exteroceptive and interoceptive stimuli and to modulate sensory, motor, and automatic processing. In terms of relevant sensory inputs, the amygdala receives direct thalamic projections from the pulvinar and the medial geniculate nucleus, and highly processed sensory information from the anterior temporal lobe. It also receives olfactory, gustatory, and visceral inputs via the olfactory bulb and the nucleus of the solitary tract. These latter inputs are thought to provide information about the positive or negative reinforcing properties of stimuli, or their biological value. In humans, amygdalar lesions can produce a general reduction of emotional responses and, specifically, a selective deficit in the recognition of fearful facial expressions [46, 50].

Together, these studies are consistent with a crucial role for the amygdala in detecting and responding to threatening situations. More generally, some studies have demonstrated that the human amygdala plays an important part in the recognition of emotion from facial expressions [51]. Moreover, the amygdala was found to have a significant role in processing emotional arousal and valence directly. Empirical data have provided details regarding impairments in recognizing facial expressions of fear in subjects with bilateral amygdala damage. However, it is not the case that bilateral amygdala damage impairs all knowledge regarding fear; rather, the knowledge that fear is highly arousing, which may be an important correlate of the ability to predict potential danger, is impaired. The amygdala may be of special importance in rapidly triggering a physiological change in response to an emotionally salient stimulus. An important component of this type of emotional response may be physiological arousal, including increases in the automatic arousal triggered by the amygdala.

Recent data from studies of human patients with amygdala damage, as well as brain imaging studies in healthy subjects, provide strong evidence that in humans and in animals the amygdala is critical for long-term declarative memory associated with emotional arousal, despite the fact that both humans and animals may experience normal emotional reactions to the material. Lesion experiments in animals suggest that the amygdala is involved in the neuromodulation of brain regions engaged in emotional learning and emotional comprehension. Specifically, many studies have demonstrated that the amygdala participates in the differential neural response to fearful and happy expressions. Analysis of the amygdala's activity with respect to other regional neural responses provided a more detailed characterization of its functional interactions and compelling evidence that this brain structure can modulate the processing of particular categories of facial expressions in the extrastriate cortex.

Finally, amygdalar activation is related to the relevance of the emotional valence of stimuli. For example, an fMRI study reported increased activity in the left amygdala associated with mood shift toward sadness. The degree of negative mood change was associated with the extent of left amygdalar activation. Another factor that was explored was the effect of emotion discrimination condition, in which the limbic response was modulated by both task (to discriminate the emotional valence of faces or other nonemotional features) and attentional demand [52, 53].

10.4 Left and Right Hemispheres in Facial Comprehension

Facial perception is also strongly influenced by the lateralization effect. The idea that the brain's two hemispheres have different functions has fascinated researchers since the last century [54]. Indeed, numerous studies, employing diverse methodologies, have examined hemispheric specialization in the perception of emotional information conveyed by different channels of communication. In parallel with the facial channel, the most frequently used measures for the vocal channel were ear differences in response to the dichotic presentation of emotionally intoned verbal and nonverbal material. For the facial channel, the most frequently used measures are visual field differences in response to tachistoscopic presentation of facial emotion and hemispace advantage.

Research on hemispheric asymmetry has benefited from of the many different instruments that can be used to draw inferences about the role of each cerebral hemisphere in the control of behavior. These include the ERP technique, magnetoencephalography, and PET. Moreover, we can distinguish between two different types of studies: those in brain-damaged patients and those in normal subjects. For the former, two special categories of patients have been of particular importance in the study of hemispheric asymmetry. The first consists of epileptic patients whose cerebral hemispheres have become disconnected (split-brain patients). These individuals are ideal for examining the respective competence of each cerebral hemisphere. The second consists of hemispherectomized individuals, i.e., those in whom one hemisphere has been ablated as a result of massive damage that disturbed the functioning of the intact hemisphere. The observation that, in some subjects, a single hemisphere can sustain nearly all major cognitive functions at a level of efficiency comparable to that in normal subjects, with two intact hemispheres, is a clear illustration that cerebral lateralization of function is a developmental process, during which the two hemispheres normally interact in distributing and acquiring their respective competencies.

Studies of the brain-behavior relationship have also explored the respective contribution of the intact cerebral hemispheres to cognitive functions. A recent approach to uncovering the functional organization of the normal human brain consists of PET measurements of local changes in cerebral blood flow (CBF) during the performance of mental tasks. The introduction of paired-image subtraction and intersubject averaging has enhanced the sensitivity of PET in measuring regional CBF and has opened the way to the study of anatomic-functional correlations of higher-order cognitive processing.

An interesting example of the application of these methodologies is the study of selected groups of brain-damaged patients: prosopagnosic, hemispherectomized, and split-brain patients. For example, some investigations have revealed a large number of prosopagnosia patients in whom cerebral injury is restricted to the right hemisphere. The fact that prosopagnosia can result from unilateral right hemisphere damage strongly suggests a crucial role for the right hemisphere in facial processing and may even indicate that this hemisphere is both necessary and sufficient to sustain facial recognition abilities. The examination of hemispherectomized patients has suggested a functional equivalence of the hemispheres in facial processing, as facial processing deficits have not been reported in any of these patients. Hemispheric equivalence in facial processing is also suggested by research on split-brain patients. Specifically, both the right and the left hemispheres were found to be capable of recognizing faces and associating a name with a face, and that each could do so without the contribution of the other. Thus, findings from these three categories of patients support the view of a functional equivalence of the cerebral hemispheres in facial processing.

Nonetheless, the findings with respect to the contribution of the cerebral hemispheres to facial processing are conflicting. Whereas facial processing impairments occur nearly exclusively in patients with lesions in the right hemisphere, evidence from split-brain and hemispherectomized patients suggests the functional equivalence of the two hemispheres with respect to facial processing or, at least, that destruction of areas in both hemispheres is necessary to produce a complete inability to process faces. Two theories have been offered to explain these discrepancies and the hemispheric differences in facial expression comprehension: (1) dominance of the right hemisphere in emotion perception [55], which may lead to the increase in the perceived emotional intensity of the right half of the face and (2) a valence approach, according to which negative and positive emotions are lateralized to different hemispheres [56]. We discuss the two different hypotheses in the next paragraph, taking into account recent empirical evidence.

10.4.1 Asymmetry of Emotional Processing

The focus of a recent experimental paradigm of analysis was *approach-related positive emotion* and *withdrawal-related emotion*. In experiments carried out by Davidson [57], subjects were offered stimuli designed to induce approach-related positive emotion and withdrawal-related negative emotions. Happiness and amusement were the positive, approach-related emotions and disgust was the negative, withdrawal-related emotion. Brain electrical activity was recorded from the left and right frontal, central, anterior temporal, and parietal regions (see Fig. 10.4). An EEG was acquired during periods of happy and disgusted facial expressions and the power at different frequency bands was calculated. The authors hypothesized that right-sided anterior activation would be more strongly associated with periods of disgust and left-sided activation with happy periods. Indeed, disgust was associated with less alpha power (more activation) in the right frontal lead whereas happiness was associated with less alpha power in the left frontal lead.

Nevertheless, there have been considerable inconsistencies in the results of divided-visual-field studies, including facial studies. The first problem is that facial processing was considered as a single process. For example, no distinction was made between familiar and unfamiliar faces, and most studies involved the presentation of unfamiliar faces. However, a distinction between the processing of familiar and unfamiliar faces has received support from PET studies, as different cortical areas are activated depending on the category of faces presented. If one accepts the results of divided-visual-field studies of facial processing, it would seem justified to conclude that both cerebral hemispheres are equipped with the necessary structures to carry out facial discrimination and recognition, as well as processing of the visually derived semantic properties of faces. This conclusion relies on the fact that one can always find at least one study showing that the left or right hemisphere is the more competent one at any of the operations that have been examined. There is, however, one exception: there is no study indicating that the left hemisphere is better than the right in the delayed matching of faces, whereas there are several studies showing better left hemisphere ability to identify famous or well-known faces [58]. This might suggest a special role for the right hemisphere in the initial storage of facial information, but an equal ability of the cerebral hemispheres to access stored facial information. Most experiments using accuracy as the main dependent variable have established right hemisphere superiority, whereas some results have suggested a role for the left hemisphere in the latency of response for faces. This makes it difficult to draw definite conclusions from these studies.

The main theories about the asymmetry of emotional processing can be grouped into four general categories, summarized as follows:

1. the right hemisphere has a general superiority (or dominance) over the left hemisphere with respect to various aspects of emotional behavior;
2. the two hemispheres have a complementary specialization in the control of different aspects of mood. In particular, the left hemisphere is considered to be dominant for positive emotions and the right hemisphere for negative emotions;
3. the right hemisphere is dominant for emotional expression in a manner analogous to that of the dominance of the left hemisphere for language;
4. the right hemisphere is dominant for the perception of emotion-related cues, such as nuances of facial expression, posture, and prosody.

The studies reported thus far have not led to a clear resolution as to which theory best fits the available data. Some of the difficulties are due to the heterogeneous experimental situations. Kolb and Taylor [59] stated that it is unlikely that the brain evolved an asymmetric control of emotional behavior. Rather, it seems more likely that, although there may be some asymmetry in the neural control of emotion, the observed asymmetries are largely a product of the asymmetric control of other functions, such as the control of movement and language.

Moreover, the *valence hypothesis* assumed in its first version that right and left hemisphere specialization for, respectively, negative and positive emotions is independent of processing modes. The degree of pleasantness would be critical to the hemispheric involvement in emotions: withdrawal is connected with the right hemisphere, whereas approach behavior is connected with the left hemisphere [60]. Successively it was proposed that hemispheric specialization according to valence is observed only for the expression of emotion, whereas the perception of emotion is assumed to be located in right posterior regions (for a discussion of this issue, see also Chapter 11). Nonetheless, various investigations have proposed that the right hemisphere is dominant in the expression and perception of emotion, regardless of valence. What is the evidence for this assumption? First, emotional processing is known to involve strategies (nonverbal, integrative, holistic) and functions (pattern perception, visuospatial organization) that are specific to the right hemisphere. By contrast, the left hemisphere is more involved in activation and focal attention. A second point is that the right hemisphere is more strongly linked to subcortical structures fundamental for arousal and intention. Due to their respective processing features, the right hemisphere is more prone to nonverbal (emotional) processing and the left to verbal (linguistic) processing.

10.5 The Universe of Emotions: Different Brain Networks for Different Emotions?

10.5.1 Emotional Valence and the Arousal of Facial Expressions

Previous studies on the impairment of facial-expression recognition suggested category-specific deficits for the decoding of emotional expressions (e.g., fear and not happiness) after brain injury involving the amygdala. Moreover, emotionally expressive faces have been shown to have an influence on a number of processes. The viewing of affective stimuli elicits emotional reactions in self-report, autonomic, and somatic measures. Depending on these emotions, there are differential effects on sympathetic dermal and on cardiovascular reactions [61], facial EMG [62], skin reaction [63], and amygdalar activation in fMRI studies and in ERPs [34]. In addition, the human brain differentiates between pleasant and unpleasant stimuli earlier than was previously thought and both hemispheres are able to perform this differentiation [64].

An important and currently questioned issue is the effect of the emotional valence of the stimulus on ERP correlates. The findings of previous research have pointed out a modulation of late deflections of ERP as a function of facial "motivational significance" [65]. Specifically, an ERP deflection of greater magnitude characterizes the response to emotionally salient stimuli (unpleasant compared to neutral). This effect has been theoretically related to motivated attention, in which motivationally relevant stimuli naturally arouse and direct attentional resources [66].

More generally, in the appraisal model each emotional expression represents the subject's response to a particular kind of significant event, either harmful or beneficial, that motivates coping activity [67, 68]. Negative high-arousal emotions (such as anger, fear, and surprise) are expressions of a situation perceived as threatening and of the subject's inability to confront the event. By contrast, negative low-arousal emotions (such as sadness) represent a negative situation and, at the same time, the subject's deactivation of an active response. Finally, positive high-arousal emotions (such as happiness) express the effectiveness of managing an external stimulus, and its positive value. For this reason, facial expressions are an important key to explaining the emotional situation and they can produce different reactions in a viewer. As a whole, the "significance" of emotional expressions for the subject and their low/high threatening power should influence both the physiological (e.g., the response to the stimulus in terms of skin conductance or arousal) and the cognitive (mental response in terms of evaluation) levels, with corresponding ERP responses.

Thus, a main question of current research concerns the effect of the type of emotions on facial processing [11]. Recent neuropsychological and, specifically, ERP data have been interpreted as indicating that emotional perception, and especially the perception of facial expressions, is organized in a modular fashion, with distinct neural circuitry subserving individual emotions. Nevertheless, only a few studies have examined the range of "basic" emotions or distinguished possible differential cortical activation as a function of the emotions. Moreover, those that analyzed face-specific brain potentials did not exhaustively explore the emotional content of faces and the effect on ERPs [26]. In some cases, only a limited number of emotions was considered, usually a comparison of one positive and one negative emotion, such as sadness and happiness. In an investigation of the specific effect of different facial expressions, carried out by Herrmann and colleagues [27], expressions with three different emotional valences (sad, happy, and neutral) were compared.

10.5.2 N200 ERP Effect in Emotional Face Decoding

Our recent study was designed to clarify the issue as to whether the face-specific brain potential is modified by the emotional valence of facial stimuli. We extended the range of emotional expressions, considering two features, arousal (high *vs* low) and the hedonic (positive *vs* negative) valence of the facial stimulus. The main question was whether the "salience value" of facial expressions has an effect on stimulus elaboration, and whether it is revealed by ERP variations. How can these effects of motivation and salience of emotional facial expressions on ERPs be explained? The appraisal of motivational relevance is essential because it determines to what extent a stimulus or situation furthers or endangers an organism's survival or adaptation to a given environment [69]. The implications of the event for the well-being of the organism take center stage, involving primary appraisal, according to Lazarus [70]. For example, an event is relevant if it threatens one's livelihood or even one's survival. This dimension occupies a central position in appraisal theories. Smith and Lazarus [71] used "importance" and "perceived obstacle," while Scherer [72] proposed "concern relevance." Relevance as a continuous dimension, from low to high, may depend on the number of goals or needs affected and their relative priority in the hierarchy.

In line with this perspective, we hypothesized that, if ERP variations are useful markers of the cognitive processes underlying emotion encoding, there must be significant differences between the two categories (high/low) of salient emotions. Thus, ERP variations are expected to be affected by the emotional content of the facial expression. Consistent with the "functional model," we proposed that subjects are more emotionally involved by a high-threatening negative emotion (i.e., fear) than by a low-threatening positive emotion (happiness), that they might have a more intense emotional reaction while viewing a negative highly-involving (highly salient, i.e., fear) than a negative less-involving (less salient, i.e., sadness) emotion [73]. Consequently, the level of attention may change as a function of a face's salience value, such that ERP measures can become a significant marker of the increased involvement and attention addressed to salient stimuli.

The ERP profiles observed in the emotional face-expression decoding showed a significant negative deflection for each of the five emotional face expressions (Fig. 10.5). The deflection peaked at approximately 230 ms. However, a similar deflection was not observed for neutral faces. We hypothesized that this deflection was strictly related to the decoding of emotion facial expressions, as revealed in previous ERP studies [74]. In order to evaluate more precisely the frontal-posterior distribution of peak variations, a more restricted comparison was carried out, considering the anterior and posterior location (anterior *vs* posterior) of electrode sites. The data showed, in addition to the main effect of type of emotion, a significant interaction between effect type and localization, with a more posteriorly distributed peak for each of the emotional expressions, but not in the case of neutral stimuli. This more posterior distribution of the peak for all of the expressions is in line with previous results, in which emotional visual area activation covering a broad range of the occipitotemporal cortices was reported [75].

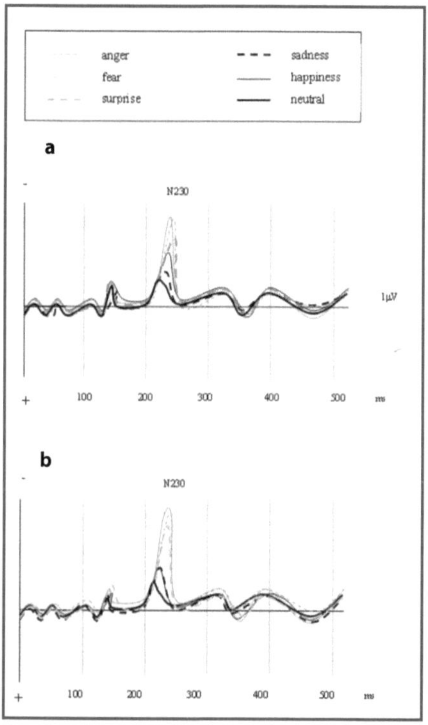

Fig. 10.5 (**a**) Grand-averaged ERP waveforms at the Fz electrode site for the six facial expressions; (**b**) Grand-averaged waveforms at the Pz electrode

10

Nevertheless, we observed that the negative ERP variation differed among the five emotions in terms of peak amplitude. Indeed, whereas there were no differences between anger, fear, and surprise, happiness and sadness had a more positive peak than the three high-arousal expressions. The different profiles of the ERPs as a function of the emotional valence of the stimulus may indicate the sensibility of the negative-wave variation N230 to the "emotional" value of the expressions [76]. Very similar potentials, with identical early latency and amplitude, were observed for happy and sad expressions, differentiated from the negative high-arousal emotions (fear, anger, and surprise).

Our results allowed us to extend the range of emotions and to explore the effect of several parameters on ERP variation. Two major parameters appear to affect the ERP profile: high/low arousal and the negative/positive value of the emotional expression. Specifically, not only may negative emotions (like anger) induce a stronger reaction within the subject than positive emotions (like happiness), with more intense emotional response, experienced emotional intensity may increase while viewing a negative high-arousal emotion (anger) but decrease while viewing a negative low-arousal emotional expression (sadness). This assumption is strengthened by the finding of the corresponding behavioral responses of the subject: fear, anger, and surprise elicited negative intense feelings whereas happiness and, especially, sadness were less involving and less intense. Therefore, it can be assumed that as a function of arousal (from higher to lower) and hedonic value (from negative to positive) emotional expressions are distributed along a continuum, as are the subjects' emotional response to them. This fact is reflected by ERP variations, with an increasing negativity of the N230.

We propose that the induction of emotional processes within a subject by the perception of emotionally expressive faces is a powerful instrument in the detection of emotional states in others and provides the basis for one's own reactions. From an evolutionary point of view, negative emotions appear to be most prominent as a human safeguard. Specifically, they facilitate the survival of the species, and the immediate and appropriate response to emotionally salient (threat-related) stimuli confers an "adaptive" value upon them.

References

1. Balconi M (2008) Emotional face comprehension. Neuropsychological perspectives. Nova Science, Hauppauge, New York
2. Ekman P (1982) Emotion in the human face, 2nd ed. Cambridge University Press, New York
3. Keltner D, Ekman P (2003) Introduction: expression of emotion. In: Davidson RJ, Scherer KR, HH Goldsmith (eds) Handbook of affective sciences, Series in affective science. Oxford University Press, Oxford, pp 411-414
4. Russell JA (1997) Reading emotions from and into faces: resurrecting a dimensional-contextual perspective. In: Russell JA, Fernández-Dols JM (eds) The psychology of facial expression. Cambridge University Press, Cambridge, pp 295-320

5. Ellsworth PC (1991) Some implications of cognitive appraisal theories of emotion. In: Strongman KT (ed) International review of studies of emotion. Wiley, New York, pp 143-161
6. Izard CE (1994) Innate and universal facial expressions: evidence from developmental cross-cultural research. Psychol Bull 115:288-299
7. Izard CE, Youngstrom EA, Fine SE et al (2006) Emotions and developmental psychopathology. In: Cicchetti D, Cohen DJ (eds) Developmental psychopathology, vol 1: Theory and method (2nd ed.). John Wiley & Sons, Hoboken, pp 244-292
8. Russell JA, Bachorowski JA, Fernández-Dols JM (2003) Facial and vocal expressions of emotions. Annu Rev Psychol 54: 359-349
9. Balconi M, Lucchiari C (2005) Morphed facial expressions elicited a N400 ERP effect. A cerebral domain-specific semantic module. Scan J Psychol 4:467-474
10. Balconi M, Lucchiari C (2005). ERP (Event-related potentials) related to normal and morphed emotional faces. The Journal of Psychology. Interdisciplinary and Applied 2:176-192
11. Balconi M, Pozzoli U (2003) Face-selective processing and the effect of pleasant and unpleasant emotional expressions on ERP correlates. Int J Psychophysiol 49:67-74
12. Smith CA, Scott HS (1998) A Componential approach to the meaning of facial expressions. In: Russell JA, Fernández-Dols JM (eds) The psychology of facial expression. Cambridge University Press, Cambridge, pp 229-254
13. Frijda NH (1994) Emotions are functional, most of the time. In: Ekman P, Davidson RJ (eds) The nature of emotion: fundamental questions. Oxford University Press, New York, pp 112-122
14. Fridlund SJ (1991) Sociality of solitary smiling: potentiation by an implicit audience. J Pers Soc Psychol 60:229-240.
15. Widen SC, Russell JA (2003) A closer look at preschoolers' freely produced labels for facial expressions. Developmental Psychol 39 114-128
16. Tomasello M, Call J (1997) Primate cognition. Oxford University Press, Oxford
17. Erickson K, Schulkin J (2003) Facial expressions of emotion: a cognitive neuroscience perspective. Brain Cognition 52:52-60
18. Bruce V, Young AW (1998) A theoretical perspective for understanding brain recognition. In: Young AW (ed) Face and mind. Oxford University Press, Oxford, pp 96-131
19. Bentin S, Deouell LY (2000) Structural encoding and identification in face processing: ERP evidence for separate mechanisms. Cognitive Neuropsychol 17:35-54
20. Posamentier MT, Abdi H (2003) Processing faces and facial expressions. Neuropsychol Rev 13:113-143
21. Haxby JV, Hoffman EA, Gobbini MI (2000) The distributed human neural system for face perception. Trends Cognitive Sci 4:223-233
22. Bernstein LJ, Beig S, Siegenthaler AL, Grady CL (2002) The effect of encoding strategy of the neural correlates of memory for faces. Neuropsychologia 40:86-98
23. Kanwisher N, McDermott J, Chun MM (1997) The fusiform face area: a module in human extrastriate cortex specialized for face perception. J Neurosci 17:4302-4311
24. Grelotti DG, Gauthier I, Schultz RT (2002) Social interest and the development of cortical face specialization: what autism teaches us about face processing. Devel Psychobiol 40:213-225
25. Adolphs R, Damasio H, Tranel D, Damasio AR (1996) Cortical systems for the recognition of emotion in facial expressions. J Neurosci 16:7678-7687
26. Eimer M, McCarthy RA (1999) Prosopagnosia and structural encoding of faces: evidence from event-related potentials. Neuroreport 10:255-259
27. Herrman MJ, Aranda D, Ellgring H et al (2002) Face-specific event-related potential in humans is independent from facial expression. Int J Psychophisiol 45:241-244

28. Caldara R, Thut G, Servoir P et al (2003) Face versus non-face object perception and the "other-race" effect: aspatio-temporal event-related potential study. Clinical Neurophysiol 114:515-528
29. Eimer M (2000) Attentional modulations of event-related brain potentials sensitive to faces. Cognitive Neuropsychol 17:103-116
30. Bentin S, Deouell LY (2000) Structural encoding and identification in face processing: ERP evidence for separate mechanisms. Cognitive Neuropsychol 17:35-54
31. Rossion B, Gauthier I, Tarr MJ et al (2000) The N170 occipito-temporal component is delayed and enhanced to inverted faces but not to inverted objects: an electrophysiological account of face-specific processes in the human brain. Neuroreport 11:69-74
32. Jemel B, George, Olivares E et al (1999) Event-related potentials to structural familiar face incongruity processing. Psychophysiology 36:437-452
33. Holmes A, Vuilleumier P, Eimer M (2003) The processing of emotional facial expressions is gated by spatial attention: evidence from event-related brain potentials. Cognitive Brain Res 16:174-184
34. Junghöfer M, Bradley MM, Elbert TR, Lang PJ (2001) Fleeting images: a new look at early emotion discrimination. Psychophysiology 38:175-178
35. Olivares EI, Iglesias J, Bobes MA (1998) Searching for face-specific long latency ERPs: a topographic study of effects associated with mismatching features. Cognitive Brain Res 7:343-356
36. Balconi M, Pozzoli U (2005) Comprehending semantic and grammatical violations in Italian. N400 and P600 comparison with visual and auditory stimuli. J Psycholinguist Res 34:71-99
37. Kutas M, Federmeier KD (2001) Electrophysiology reveals semantic memory use in language comprehension. Trends Cognitive Sci 4: 463-470
38. Balconi M (2002) Neuropsicologia della comunicazione [Neuropsycholgy of communication]. In: Anolli L (ed) Manuale di psicologia della comunicazione [Handbook of the psychology of communication]. Il Mulino, Bologna, pp 85-125
39. Huddy V, Schweinberger SR, Jentzsch I, Burton AM (2003) Matching faces for semantic information and names: an event-related brain potentials study. Cognitive Brain Res 17:314-326
40. Münte TF, Brack M, Groother O et al (1998) Brain potentials reveal the timing of face identity and expression judgments. Neurosci Res 30:25-34
41. LeDoux JE (1996) The emotional brain: the misterious underpinning of emotional life. Simon and Schuster, New York
42. Philips ML, Young AW, Senior C et al (1997) A specific neural substrate for perceiving facial expressions of disgust. Nature 389:495-498
43. Allison T, Puce A, Spencer D, McCarthy G (1999) Electrophysiological studies of human face perception. I: Potentials generated in occipitotemporal cortex by face and non-face stimuli. Cereb Cortex 9:415-430
44. Schultz RT, Gauthier I, Klin A et al (2000) Abnormal ventral temporal cortical activity during face discrimination among individuals with autism and Asperger syndrome. Arch Gen Psychiat 57:331-340
45. Teunisse JP, de Gelder B (2001) Impaired categorical perception of facial expressions in high-functioning adolescents with autism. Child Neuropsychol 7:1-14
46. Adolphs R, Schul, R, Tranel D (1998) Intact recognition of facial emotion in Parkinson's disease. Neuropsychology 12:253-258
47. Adolphs R (2003) Investigating the cognitive neuroscience of social behavior. Neuropsychologia 41:119-126
48. Allison T, Puce A, McCarthy G (2000) Social perception from visual cues: role of the STS region. Trends Cognitive Sci 4:267-278

49. Davidson RJ (1994) Asymmetric brain function, affective style and psychopathology: the role of early experience and plasticity. Devel Psychopathol 6:741-758
50. Calder AJ, Burton AM, Miller P et al (2001) A principal component analysis of facial expressions. Vision Res 41:1179-1208
51. Adolphs R (1999) Social cognition and the human brain. Trends Cognitive Sci 3:469-479
52. Vuilleumier P, Schwartz S (2001) Emotional facial expressions capture attention. Neurology 56:153-158
53. Gurr B, Moffat N (2001) Psychological consequences of vertigo and the effectiveness of vestibular rehabilitation for brain injury patients. Brain Injury 15:387-400
54. Banich MT (1997) Neuropsychology. The human bases of mental function. Houghton Mifflin Company, New York
55. Borod JC (1993) Cerebral mechanisms underlying facial, prosodic, and lexical emotional expression: a review of neuropsychological studies and methodological issues. Neuropsychology 7:445-463
56. Adolphs R, Jansari A, Tranel D (2001) Hemispheric perception of emotional valence from facial expressions. Neuropsychology 15:516-524
57. Davidson RJ, Hugdahl K (1995) Brain asymmetry. The MIT Press, Cambridge, MA
58. Eimer M (1998) Does the face specific N170 component reflect the activity of a specialized eye processor? Neuroreport 9:2945-2948
59. Kolb B, Taylor L (1990) Neocortical substrates of emotional behavior. In: Stein NL, Lewenthal B, Trabasso T (eds) Psychological and biological approaches to emotion. Lawrence Erlbaum Associates, Hillsdale, pp 115-144
60. Pizzigalli D (1998) Face, word and emotional processing: electrophysiological (EEG and ERP) studies on emotions with a focus on personality. Zentralstelle der Studentenschaft, Zurich
61. Lang PJ, Greenwald MK, Bradley MM, Hamm AO (1993) Looking at pictures: affective, facial, visceral and behavioral reactions. Psychophysiology 30:261-273
62. Dimberg U (1997) Facial reactions: rapidly evoked emotional responses. J Psychophysiol, 11:115-123
63. Esteves F, Parra C, Dimberg U, Öhman A (1994) Nonconscious associative learning: pavlovian conditioning of skin conductance responses to masked fear-relevant stimuli. Psychophysiology 31:375-385
64. Pizzagalli D, Koenig T, Regard M, Lehmann D (1999) Affective attitudes to face images associated with intracerebral EEG source location before face viewing. Brain Res Cognitive Brain Res 7:371-377
65. Lang PJ, Bradley MM, Cuthbert BN (1997) Motivated attention: affect, activation, and action. In: Lang PJ, Simons RF, Balaban M (eds) Attention and orienting: sensory and motivational processes. Erlbaum, Mahwah, pp 97-135
66. Keil A, Bradley MM, Hauk O et al (2002) Large-scale neural correlates of affective picture processing. Psychophysiology 39:641-649
67. Frijda NH (1994) Emotions are functional, most of the time. In: Ekman P, Davidson RJ (eds) The nature of emotion: fundamental questions. Oxford University Press, New York, pp 112-122
68. Hamm AO, Schupp HT, Weike AI (2003) Motivational organization of emotions: autonomic change cortical responses, and reflex modulation. In: Davidson RJ, Scherer KR, Goldsmith HH (eds) Handbook of affective neurosciences. Oxford University Press, Oxford, pp 187-212
69. Ellsworth PC, Scherer KR (2003) Appraisal processes in emotion. In: Davidson RJ, Scherer KR, Goldsmith HH (eds) Handbook of affective neurosciences. Oxford University Press, Oxford, pp 572-596
70. Lazarus RS (1999) Appraisal, relational meaning, and emotion. In: Dalgleish T, Power M (eds) Handbook of cognition and emotion. Wiley, Chichester, pp 3-19

71. Smith CA, Lazarus RS (1990) Emotion and adaptation. In: Pervin LA (ed), Handbook of personality: theory and research. Guilford, New York, pp 609-637
72. Scherer KR (2001) The nature and study of appraisal: a review of the issues. In: Scherer KR, Schorr A, Johnstone T (eds) Appraisal processes in emotion: theory, methods, research. Oxford University Press, New York, pp 369-391
73. Wild B, Erb M, Bartels M (2001) Are emotions contagious? Evoked emotions while viewing emotional expressive faces: quality, quantity, time course and gender differences. Psych Res 102:109-124
74. Streit M, Wölwer W, Brinkmeyer J et al (2000) Electrophysiological correlates of emotional and structural face processing in humans. Neurosci Letters 278:13-16
75. Sato W, Takanori K, Sakiko Y, Michikazu M (2001) Emotional expression boosts early visual processing of the face: ERP reecording and its decomposition by independent component analysis. Neuroreport 12:709-714
76. Jung TP, Makeig S, Humphries C et al (2000) Removing electroencephalographic artifacts by blind source separation. Psychophysiology 37:163-178

Emotions, Attitudes and Personality: Psychophysiological Correlates

11

M. Balconi

11.1 Introduction

There is a long tradition in emotion psychology of examining facial expressions as a visible indicator of unobservable emotional processes. On the one hand, cognitive research into facial expression has pointed out the *cognitive role* of processes underlying facial decoding and their specificity compared to other cognitive mechanisms. On the other hand, theoretical paradigms of the analysis of emotions have underlined the *early emergence* of this cognitive skill during ontogenesis, as well as the *social significance* of this acquisition.

The multifunctionality of facial expressions, due to the fact that they also have nonemotional significance, introduces the issue of the *communicative* and *social meanings* of facial expressions. Among the expressive elements that contribute to the communication of emotion, facial expressions are considered as communicative cues. In other words, they are conceptualized as social tools that aid in the negotiation of social interactions. As such, they are a declaration of our trajectory in a given social interaction. The social aspect is present even when an individual is alone, since others may be present psychologically, and people talk to themselves, interact with imagined others, replay prior interactions. Thus, facial expressions serve the *social motives* of the displayer. In addition, *personality* and subjective *attitudes* and *motivations* have been implicated in facial processing, since they contribute to explaining the heterogeneous responses to emotional expressions.

M. Balconi (✉)
Department of Psychology, Catholic University of Milan, Milan, Italy

Neuropsychology of Communication. Michela Balconi (Ed.)

11.2 Facial Expression of Emotions as an Integrated Symbolic Message

Given that the communicative behavior of encoder and decoder has evolved in reciprocal fashion, an individual's emotional expression serves as a social *affordance* that evokes responses in others. Stated succinctly, facial expressions evoke emotions in others. For example, Dimberg and Öhman [1] documented that displays of anger evoke fear in decoders, and, as in infants as young as 8 months of age, overt displays of distress evoke concern as well as overt attempts to help. However, the meaning and function of such displays may not be apparent when viewed out of context [2]. Understanding how facial displays contribute to conversation and social interactions requires that we consider context in determining the nature of the display. Communicative models have focused on the study of facial action in dialogue, concluding that facial displays are *active, symbolic components* of *integrated messages* (including words, intonations, and gestures) [3].

Most facial actions in dialogue are symbolic acts; like words, they convey information from one person to the other. As *integrated message*, the combination of words, facial expressions, gestures, etc., is an important feature of conversational language. The importance of nonverbal elements such as facial expressions has been emphasized by many researchers. For example, facial expressions are synchronized with speech [4]: they can work together to create a syntax and a semantic form; also, faces engaged in dialogue move to convey meaning in conjunction with other, simultaneous symbolic acts. Consequently, it is necessary to analyze facial displays as they occur in actual social interactions, with the goal of understanding their meaning in context. Just as with words, we have to locate facial expressions in the ongoing development of the dialogue, which is built around the topic of conversation, and we must consider what is happening at the moment. Thus, the cumulative context must be considered, that is, the simultaneous occurrence of other symbolic acts, words, gestures, intonation, etc., that accompany facial action. These symbolic acts are integrated with each other to create the complete meaning.

11.3 Developmental Issues: Dimensionality in the Child's Emotional Face Acquisition

Recent empirical evidence has underlined the significance of specific dimensions in the acquisition of recognition skills by the child, lending support to the so-called dimensional approach to emotional face recognition [5]. This evidence was obtained by comparing the ability of adults *vs* infants to comprehend facial expressions of emotion and by analyzing the development of decoding abilities in infants. Additionally, the relative contributions of cognitive and neuropsychological correlates to facial comprehension ability were evaluated.

Infants show an impressive ability to recognize faces [6] but it is unclear whether the different modes of facial processing are a result of development and experience or innate. Several studies have shown that infants process configural information in faces and respond to different internal sections of faces, including single facial features. Specifically, 8-month-old infants were observed to process single facial features such as the eyes and mouth in conjunction with the facial context. Empirical data suggest that even very young infants are able to discriminate facial features interpreted by an adult as facial expressions. However, this seems to first occur at age 6–7 months while beforehand expressions are interpreted as being the same despite discriminable differences in their intensity [7].

The development of facial processing as a function of neuropsychological maturation was explored by de Haan, Pascalis, and Johnson [8]. One factor contributing to the ability to recognize expressions is maturation of the neural systems involved in recognition, since the ability to recognize facial expressions represents a selective adaptation in which specialized neural systems are created for this purpose. This finding is partly derived from studies showing that infants just a few months old are able to discriminate among different "types" of expressions. Specifically, the temporal lobe and the prefrontal cortex are involved in the perception, discrimination, and recognition of facial expression.

Both behavioral studies in humans and anatomical studies in monkeys suggested that there are developmental periods when the ability to recognize expression may change. Discrimination starts at about 3 months of age, but recognition of negative expressions may not occur until the second year. These data might be considered as the strongest evidence of an adaptive ability that has been selected through evolution. Nevertheless, the presence of dedicated neural hardware does not rule out a role for *experience* in development. For example, experience could regulate those genes related to facial-expression recognition. Thus the ability to respond at age 6–7 months to categories of expressions, rather than isolated features, may parallel the differential maturation of brain structures such as the amygdala. It is clear that the discrimination and recognition of facial expressions entails identifiable patterns of activity in the brain, with certain cells in the amygdala and areas of the anterior temporal lobe more responsive to facial stimuli than to other patterned stimuli.

It is also important to distinguish between *recognizing* and *labeling* an emotional face. Empirical analysis of behavioral measures of emotion recognition in infants and theoretical analysis of the evolutionary advantages of an emotion signaling system in the production and recognition of facial expressions suggest that, whereas children recognize specific emotions from facial expressions, their performance in labeling facial expressions is modest and improves only gradually with age [9].

Children's interpretation of emotions has been addressed methodologically in a number of ways: they have been asked to match emotional expressions with situations, to label emotional expressions, and to state which emotions arise in different situations. In a series of studies, Bullock and Russell [10] found that infants do not interpret facial expressions according to the same specific categories of emotions implied by researchers with the words sad, angry, etc., since while children interpret facial expressions they do so differently than adults. The child's earliest conceptual system for emotion is based on the dimensions of *pleasure* and *arousal* and is reflected accordingly in his or her response [11]. It could therefore be argued that the accuracy of the response varies with the emotion presented. The general result is that happiness is identified, differentiated, and labeled more consistently than other emotions, such as fear, anger, surprise, and sadness.

The means by which infants interpret facial expression of emotion and how their interpretation changes as development progresses form an interesting basis for exploring the conceptualization of emotional faces. Biological theories of emotion emphasize the evolutionary advantages of the communicative function of emotional facial expression. At the opposite end, it has been postulated that the child every aspect of the conceptual schema for emotions is learned or constructed from experience, with the underlying constraint that emotional expressions are initially perceived in terms of dimensions of pleasure-displeasure and degree of arousal. According to Bullock and Russell, facial labeling proceeds in a typical sequence of steps:

1. infants develop the ability to perceive changes in the face and voice of others. At least by the age of 6–10 months, the perceptual abilities for extracting facial features and for combining these into a pattern are in place;
2. early on, infants find meaning in facial expressions of emotion, albeit only in terms of pleasure-displeasure and degree of arousal. These meanings facilitate social interactions and guide infants' reactions to ambiguous events;
3. the child comes to expand the meanings attached to emotions by distinguishing among the situations in which they occur. Expressions that are similar in pleasure-displeasure or arousal are associated with different contexts, different outcomes, and different causes;
4. finally, from observing combinations of emotional expressions, situations, and words, the child becomes able to construct emotion scripts.

11.4 The Effect of Personality and Attitudes on Face Comprehension

Human emotions are organized in systems of appetitive or defensive motivation that mediate a range of attentional and action reflexes, presumably evolved from primitive approach and withdrawal tendencies [12]. The most pleasant affects are held to be associated with the appetitive motivation system, and unpleasant affects with defensive motivation [13]. Emotion fundamentally varies the activation of centrally organized appetitive and aversive motivational systems that have evolved to mediate the wide range of adaptive behaviors necessary for an organism struggling to survive in the physical world. Furthermore, the response to emotional stimuli is modulated by personal sensitivity to environmental emotional cues [14].

11.4.1 Appetitive *vs* Defensive Systems and the BIS and BAS Measures

The relationship between system evaluation and motive intensity on the one hand, and personal sensitivity to emotional cues on the other, determines the specific subjective response to emotional cues and in particular to facial expressions. A primary distinction among emotional events is whether they are appetitive or aversive, positive or negative, pleasant or unpleasant [13], which clearly relates to the motivational parameter of direction. Secondarily, hedonically valenced events differ in the degree to which they arouse or engage action, which in turn is related to an intensity parameter. Arousal, or intensity, is a critical factor in organizing the pattern of physiological responses in emotional reactions. Thus, two dimensions, pleasure and arousal, explain the larger part of emotional experience and subjective judgment [15]. In this view, evaluative reports of pleasure roughly serve to index which motivational system is activated by the stimulus (i.e., appetitive "pleasant" or defensive "unpleasant"), whereas judgments of arousal index the degree of activation of each motivation system.

Subjective ratings have been largely used in a vast amount of research [16] and, together with recent empirical data, have supported the hypothesis of varying degrees of activation of two (appetitive or aversive) underlying motivational systems. When activation of both systems is minimal (neither pleasant neither unpleasant), emotional arousal is low and events are generally labeled as being neutral [17]. From a motivational perspective, this suggests only a weak tendency to approach or withdraw from the stimulus. As defensive or appetitive motivation increases, both arousal and sympathetically mediated responses increase as well, indexing the requirements of increased attention and anticipated actual action (approach or avoidance; appetitive or defensive).

Moreover, behavioral and physiological responses to emotional pictures co-vary with system evaluation (pleasure/displeasure) and motive intensity (arousal) [17, 18]. The role temperament and personality play in influencing emotional responses has been confirmed by a large number of empirical studies and in both normal and pathological populations. For example, it was shown that high-anxiety trait is directly related to increased accuracy for negative emotional cues (mainly presented to the left visual field, right hemisphere) compared to low-anxiety trait [19, 20].

A prevalent view suggests that emotional construct is based on two general systems that orchestrate adaptive behavior [21, 22]. The first system functions to halt ongoing behavior while processing potential threat cues and is referred to as the *behavioral inhibition system* (BIS) [23]. The second system governs the engagement of action and is referred to as the *behavioral activation system* (BAS) [24] or the *behavioral approach system* [25]. Although the BIS/BAS model, as described by Gray [23, 25, 26], concerns behavioral regulation, researchers have recently become interested in how these constructs are manifested in individual differences and emotional attitudes. Gray's model is an attempt to explain behavioral motivational responses in general and, in particular, the generation of emotions relevant to approach and withdrawal behavior.

The BAS can thus be conceptualized as a motivational system that is sensitive to signals of reward and non-punishment, and which activates behavior accordingly. This system should thus be responsible for both approach and active behaviors, and the emotions associated with them generally induce the subject to approach the event/object that has generated the emotional response. Moreover, the BAS has been associated with feelings of optimism, happiness, and aggression [26], whereas extreme BAS levels have been linked to impulsivity disorders. Empirical evidences suggests that BAS subjects respond in great measure to positive, approach-related emotions, such as the expression of happiness and positive affect, which in turn confers the subject with a favorable behavior toward his or her environment [27]. Nevertheless, it is also possible that the BAS is responsible for negative affective responses when these are associated with a behavioral approach. Since the primary function of the BAS is approach motivation, and approach motivation may be associated with negative affect, then certain negative emotional cues, including those that generate anger, may be associated with an increased BAS profile [28]. Consistent with this idea, Corr [29] found that high BAS levels were associated with higher expectancies for rewards, and thus potentially with higher levels of frustration upon termination or reduction of the reward magnitude.

The BIS, conversely, inhibits behavior in response to stimuli that are novel, innately feared, and conditioned to be aversive. The aversive motivational system is responsive to non-reward and prevents the individual from experiencing negative or painful outcomes. Thus, the BIS is conceptualized as an attentional system that is sensitive to cues of punishment and non-reward and that functions to interrupt ongoing behavior in order to facilitate the processing of these cues in preparation for a response. "Inhibition" in the BIS framework refers to the abrogation of behavior in reaction to an expected or unexpected stimulus [30]. High BIS activation is associated with enhanced attention, arousal, vigilance and anxiety, while a very strong BIS corresponds to anxiety-related disorders [31] and a very weak BIS to primary psychopathy [32]. Gray also held that BIS functioning is responsible for the experience of negative feelings such as fear and anxiety in response to these cues.

Nevertheless, very few studies have tried to connect emotional cue comprehension with the subjective predisposition to respond to emotions, and most have not considered the impact of this predisposition on the autonomic system and central cortical activation, as determined by brain oscillations. Thus, a central question in neuropsychological and psychophysiological research concerns how individual differences in emotional processes are manifested in motivation and personality and how do they directly regulate the responses of the peripheral and central nervous systems.

11.4.2
New Directions: EEG Brain Oscillations and ERPs

Brain oscillations are a powerful tool with which to analyze the cognitive processes related to emotion comprehension [33-39]. Understanding the mechanisms by which the immense number of neurons in the human brain interact to produce higher cognitive functions is a major challenge in brain science. One of the candidate mechanisms, oscillatory neuroelectric activity, has recently attracted great interest. Event-related oscillations with a defined temporal relation to a sensory or cognitive event (classified as evoked or phase-locked to the event) are responsive to the functional mechanisms that engender these cognitive processes [40]. Nevertheless, although frequency bands have recently been investigated with respect to the various perceptive and cognitive domains, their specific role in emotion processing is unclear [41] and conflicting results have been obtained [38, 42]. It is therefore necessary to explore the significance of an ample range of frequency bands for emotional cue comprehension, in order to observe their specific relationship to arousal and attentional mechanisms.

Some researchers have used frontal EEG as a physiological method for examining the correspondence of BAS and BIS with approach *vs* avoidance orientations [43, 44]. In this respect, the impact of parameters such as threatening power and valence of the emotional cues was recently considered. Knyazev and Slobodskoj-Plusnin [45] verified that, in a reward condition, high BAS subjects experienced a higher level of arousal in response to positive stimuli than high BIS subjects, whereas in a punishment condition or in case of negative emotional cues the BAS group experienced a lower level of arousal. Changes in theta, beta, and gamma EEG bands were examined in response to variables reflecting emotional arousal. Higher scores on the drive subscale of BAS [22] produced increased theta and high-frequency band power in frontal regions in case of reward, whereas an opposite trend was observed for these frequency bands in case of punishment.

Empirical data likewise suggest that left- and right-frontal cortical activity reflects the strength of the BAS and BIS [43]. Individuals with relatively greater left-frontal activity (less alpha) have greater levels of BAS sensitivity (approach motivation) [46], whereas those with higher BIS scores show greater right-frontal activation [47]. Moreover, alpha activity in response to emotional cues was related to the lateralization effect. Thus, EEG research has confirmed the valence hypothesis in that there is a relative increase of left hemisphere activity with positive emotional stimuli [48, 49].

The recently described approach-withdrawal model of emotion regulation posits that emotional behaviors are associated with a balance of activity in left and right frontal areas of the brain that can be detected in asymmetry measurements. Resting frontal EEG asymmetry has been hypothesized to relate to appetitive (approach-related) and aversive (withdrawal-related) emotions, with heightened approach tendencies reflected in left-frontal activity and heightened withdrawal tendencies in right-frontal activity. Subjects with relatively less left-frontal than right-frontal activity exhibited larger negative affective responses to negative emotions and smaller positive affective responses to positive emotions [50]. Interesting results also have been obtained concerning specific facial emotional patterns, such as anger and fear. In particular, anger correlated positively and significantly with right alpha power and negatively with left alpha power. This lateralization effect was similarly observed by Harmon-Jones [51], who indicated the importance of the prefrontal cortex in emotional processing. The author argued that emotions with motivational tendencies are related to greater left frontal EEG activity.

The theta frequency range is known to be associated with attention and cognitive processes, and brain oscillations around 4 Hz respond to the relevance of the material being processed. More generally, this frequency band has been ascribed an "orienting" function, since synchronization occurred in the presence of a coordinated response indicating alertness, arousal, and readiness to process information [52]. By contrast, there are currently no specific data on delta-band modulation with respect to the emotional significance of the stimulus. The amplitude of the delta response is considerably increased during oddball experiments [53, 54] and varies as a function of the necessity of stimulus evaluation and memory updating. Accordingly, the delta response is likely related to signal detection and decision making.

To summarize, visually evoked brain oscillations in the alpha frequency range seem to be closely related to visual attention-involving and memory processes, and not merely to visual stimulus processing per se; they may also be directly related to the alert response of the subject [55]. The theta frequency range is likely associated with attention and cognitive processes, the relevance of the material being processed, and the degree of attention in visual stimuli. Finally, the delta band is mainly related to decision-making processes and to updating functions.

What remains to be determined is whether a single brain operation or psychological function for emotion decoding can be assigned to a certain type of oscillatory activity. In a recent study, we explored functional correlates of brain oscillations with regard to emotional face processing. The results emphasized the importance of distributed oscillatory networks in a specific frequency range (between 1 and 12 Hz). A critical issue in current research is the variability of frequency bands inside a known time interval, especially one that has been found to be discriminant in emotional processing, i.e., the temporal window around 200 ms latency. Based on the theory that each oscillation represents multiple functions and that these are selectively distributed in the brain in the form of parallel processing systems, then oscillatory neural assemblies can be considered with respect to a well-known event-related potential (ERP) component, the N200 effect.

An effect of oscillatory neural assembly on ERPs is likely, since their intrinsic relationship is consistent with the current paradigm of cognitive psychophysiology [56]. Accordingly, there may be an effect of brain oscillation synchronous activity on ERP correlates as well. It is reasonable to assume that the oscillatory activity of the brain is a valid index of cognitive processing and that there are multivariate relations between different sets of phenomena such as event-related oscillations (EROs) and ERPs.

Finally, in terms of the central nervous system's mechanisms for mediating emotional facial stimulus, the cortical localization of these mechanisms in the scalp remains to be determined. A specific neural mechanism can be assumed to be dedicated to emotion comprehension, since previous studies found that a posterior cortical site is activated during emotional face comprehension [57-59]. Specifically, ERP studies have shown a more posteriorly distributed peak for emotional expressions than for neutral expressions. Thus, the cortical distributions of brain oscillations can be explored to test their resemblance to ERP localization.

11.5 Specialization of the Right Hemisphere in Facial Expressions?

Several channels are used to express nonverbal signals, including facial expression, tone of voice, and gestures. Empirical research has typically led to the conclusion that the right hemisphere is specialized for nonverbal behavior. Compared to patients with left-hemisphere lesions, patients with right-hemisphere lesions in parietal regions are significantly impaired in comprehending emotional tone of voice. Patients with right-hemisphere brain damage also perform more poorly than patients with left hemisphere damage under three specific conditions: (1) when trying to discriminate between emotional faces and attempting to name emotional scenes; (2) when matching emotional expressions; and (3) when grouping both pictorially presented and written emotional scenes and faces.

The right hemisphere plays a special role in understanding emotional information, as shown by many studies that included neurologically intact participants as well. For example, using a divided visual field technique, researchers found a left visual field (right hemisphere) advantage on tasks that require participants to discriminate among emotional expressions of faces, to remember emotionally expressive faces, and to match an emotional face to a spoken word [60]. Other studies have used a paradigm involving face chimeras, composed of two half-faces spliced together to make a whole face. One half of the face expresses one emotion (happiness) and the other half another emotion (sadness). Generally, right-handed people judge a face as happier when the smile appears in their left visual field or left hemifield, which suggest that the information is judged as more emotionally salient when it is received by the right hemisphere. These results have been interpreted to mean that the processing of emotional faces preferentially engages the right hemisphere.

However, the left hemisphere is not without a role in interpreting emotion. In fact, the ability to understand emotional information depends upon a knowledge base in which nonverbal information about the meaning of emotion (nonverbal affect lexicon) is stored. This ability contrasts with the ability to process another type of emotional information, i.e., the labeling of emotions, and to understand the link between certain situations and specific emotions (emotional semantics). Safer and Leventhal [61] proposed a task to rate the emotionality of passages that vary in both emotional tone of voice and emotional content. Sometimes the emotional content was consistent with the emotional tone of voice, whereas at other times it was inconsistent. The passages were presented to either the left ear or the right ear. The results showed that participants who attended to the left ear based their ratings of emotionality on tone of voice, whereas those who attended to the right ear based their ratings on the content of the passages.

An issue that remains to be explored is whether comprehending emotional information is merely a specific example of a complex perceptual task involving relational information, rather than a distinct process for which the right hemisphere is specialized. In fact, face perception is a visuo-spatial task that involves a configuration of features organized in a particular pattern relative to one another. Perhaps no unique right-hemisphere mechanism exists for processing emotional expression; instead, maybe this hemisphere engages the same mechanism that would be called upon to recognize a face or to organize a spatial pattern into a conceptual whole. A common approach is to infer the presence of separate systems or modules by the demonstration of dissociations [62]. If two tasks depend on a common region of the brain, damage to that region will presumably interfere with the performance of both tasks. Even more interesting is the case in which the opposite dissociation is observed (double dissociation).

Many examples of dissociation between the ability to recognize a face and the ability to interpret a facial emotion exist and they suggest that the right hemisphere has a separate specialization for processing emotional information above and beyond the stimuli, such as faces, upon which that emotional information is conveyed. Cases have been reported in which patients with prosopagnosia were able to identify facial emotions. Other patients could recognize faces but could not identify facial emotion. Research examining face *vs* emotional perception in neurologically intact individuals reached similar conclusions. A number of studies found that when emotional and non-emotional faces are projected by means of a divided visual field, participants exhibited a greater left visual field advantage for emotional faces than for non-emotional faces. Thus, we can ask whether all emotion is specialized to the *right hemisphere*, or is the *left hemisphere* specialized for positive emotion and the right hemisphere for negative emotion? It is clear that just because a hemisphere is associated with a particular emotional state it is not necessarily specialized to process information corresponding to that emotion [63].

11.5.1 Lateralization Effect and Valence

Right hemisphere superiority for discriminating emotional faces has been shown by *affect discrimination* [64] and was confirmed in studies in which patients with right-hemisphere lesions were less able to recognize facial expressions than patients with left-hemisphere lesions [65, 66]. Moreover, ERP and functional magnetic resonance imaging (fMRI) studies support right hemisphere specialization for the processing of facial emotions [67, 68]. In the *expression of emotions*, there appears to be facial asymmetry, with the left side of the face (right-controlled) being emotionally more expressive [69, 70]. Also, a reduced ability for facial emotional expression in patients with right-hemisphere damage was identified.

Nevertheless, other models have been formulated regarding the lateralization effect, offering alternative explanations of hemispheric differences. According to the *valence model*, and in contrast to the *right-hemisphere model*, cortical differences between the two hemispheres are attributable to the positive *vs* negative valence of emotions [71, 72]. The valence model was tested in terms of the expression and perception of emotions, as well as emotional experience. It proposes that the right hemisphere is specialized for negative emotions and the left hemisphere for positive emotions. A study found that reaction times were shorter for happy faces presented to the right visual field (left hemisphere) [73], whereas negative affective faces are identified more rapidly when presented within the right visual field [74]. Generally, right-hemisphere injury prevents these patients from processing more negative *vs* positive expressions. Some EEG studies have supported the valence hypothesis: a relative increase of left-hemisphere activity was found with positive emotional states [48], but opposite results have been reported as well (for example, [75]).

Interesting experimental results were obtained regarding specific emotional patterns. In particular, sadness correlated positively with right alpha power and negatively with left alpha power, whereas happiness was mainly related to left-side activation [76]. For other emotions, such as anger, the findings were heterogeneous. Overall, lateralized electrophysiological parameters (decreased alpha power EEG) measured during the recollection of events associated with anger increased within the right hemisphere [77]. However, once again, opposing results have been collected in other studies [78], in which increased left frontal cortical activity was associated with anger [28], and increased left frontal activity and decreased right frontal activity were associated with trait anger [79] and state anger [28].

The valence model and the right-hemisphere model make different previsions on the lateralization of the emotion of anger. Furthermore, in the *approach-withdrawal model* anger is predicted to be associated with relatively greater left frontal activity, whereas in the valence model right frontal activity would be higher. This difference is due to the fact that in the approach-withdrawal model anger is considered as an approach motivational tendency with a negative valence and not as a negative emotion per se. Approach motivation would be correlated with increased left frontal cortical activity regardless of the valence of the emotional cue. These variable and at conflicting trends require deeper analysis in order to explain the contrasting results that have been reported. Moreover, it is worth noting that many studies did not systematically manipulate the crossing effect of emotional arousal and valence in their design. For this reason, their results may have been implicitly affected by high/low arousal distinction.

11.5.2
Emotional Type Effect Explained by the "Functional Model"

As discussed above, the lateralization effect in facial expression perception may be explained by the right-side, the valence, or the approach-withdrawal model, and a large amount of data have been furnished in support of one *vs* another. Some of the contrasting results remain to be clarified in terms of the real significance of each emotion with respect to its functional value. In this functional assessment of emotional expression, people adopt a behavior that is functional to their coping activity [80, 81] which in turn determines the significance of an emotional situation, since it orients the subject's behavior as a function of his or her expectancies about successfully acting on the situation/external context. In fact, whereas some negative emotional expressions, such as anger and sadness, are generated by negative, aversive situations, the coping potential may introduce differences in subjective response as a function of how people appraise their ability to cope with the aversive situation. From this perspective, anger may be appraised as a negative but also as an active emotion, in which case it would arouse approach motivation.

In this view, facial expressions are an important key to explaining the emotional situation and, consequently, they can produce different reactions in a viewer. As a whole, the significance of emotional expressions for the subject (in terms of their high/low averseness, valence, and the individual's coping potential for the corresponding emotion) is their influence at the physiological and cognitive levels, as well as their correspondence to EEG modulation. Emotional expressions can thus be seen as being distributed along a continuum based on the motivational significance of the emotional cue in terms of averseness (from higher to lower), hedonic value (from negative to positive), and coping potential [38].

11.5.3 Recent Empirical Evidences: Frequency Band Analysis and BIS/BAS

Our research has shown a greater right- than left-side activation for certain negative emotions and a reverse tendency (left- more than right-side) for the positive emotion of happiness [82]. The absence of significant left-side activation in response to negative faces and, conversely, right-side activation to positive faces reinforced these results. Thus, negative emotional stimuli were able to induce a more intense response by the right hemisphere, whereas positive stimuli were responsible for a more accentuated left-hemisphere response. A possible explanation for these findings is that the right hemisphere selectively attends to negative facial stimuli whereas the left hemisphere shows increased attention toward positive faces. In fact, studies applied to normal or clinical populations have found hemispheric differences as a function of positive *vs* negative emotions. These differences were attributed to the facility with which the two hemispheres identify specific emotional types [71]. For example, as noted above, reaction times were shorter for happy faces shown within the right visual field (left hemisphere) and for sad faces presented within the left visual field (right hemisphere) [83].

A critical point of interest here is the fact that right-frontal prevalence was found for all negative emotional faces but not for sadness. This result is in contrast to the right-side negative hypothesis and is not accounted for by other empirical investigations. Nevertheless, it should be noted that some EEG researchers, investigating the positive-negative distinction, have found opposite patterns of activation. Based on these data, a more exhaustive paradigm of analysis may be adopted, one that takes into account both the valence (positive *vs* negative) and the degree of averseness (high *vs* low) of the emotional stimuli. The circumflex model, discussed in detail below, is able to explain frontal-right facilitation for some emotional types, that is, negative, high arousal, aversive emotional expressions, and frontal-right inhibition for emotions characterized by less arousing power, with a concomitantly reduced significance in producing a lateralization effect. Although we have not directly tested the arousing power and averseness of each emotional face, previous studies have underlined the differential impact of anger, fear, and disgust on facial expressions compared to sadness [59, 83].

The *circumflex model* predicts that the structure of emotional expression and comprehension is related to a roughly circular order in a two-dimensional space, the axes of which could be interpreted as pleasure-displeasure and arousal-sleepiness. The two orthogonal axes allow for a clear categorization of emotion perception, subdividing the entire emotional universe as a function of the arousal response produced by emotional patterns in addition to the negative/positive value of these patterns. In general, it is possible that higher aversive and arousing stimuli (fear, anger, disgust and surprise) induce a clear cortical lateralization within the right side, whereas sadness generates a less significant response. Moreover, a particular effect is related to anger, which induces a greater increase in right than in left cortical activity. Previous studies on anger experience found an opposite pattern, with a greater activation of the left than the right hemisphere [84]. This result is consistent with the position that anger is an approach motivational tendency with negative emotional valence, and, more generally, that left frontal activity is associated with approach motivation, regardless of the valence (positive *vs* negative) of the emotion. In the circumflex model, right cortical activation could be explained by taking into account the fact that, in most cases, an angry face generates a fear response in the viewer, such that the anger profile could be similar to that of fear. An additional point is related to the subjective response to emotional cues—as a function of BAS and BIS—which may have an effect on hemispheric differences. It was previously shown that, in general, people with higher BAS scores have an increased left-frontal activation, whereas those with higher BIS scores have greater right-frontal activation. Moreover, individuals with high BAS and BIS scores experience more positive and negative affect, respectively, during everyday experience [85] and exhibit greater sensitivity to positive (BAS) and negative (BIS) cues [86].

These findings are consistent with data suggesting that greater left-frontal and right-frontal activity is associated with, respectively, a more positive and more negative evaluation of equivalent stimuli. In BIS subjects the right-frontal side was more responsive to negative faces and an increased response to happiness was not detected on the left side, thus indicating a substantial equivalence of left/right side in the elaboration of positive facial expressions. Conversely, BAS subjects were more responsive to the positive facial expression of happiness, with increased activity in the left-frontal area. An interesting and unexpected result was obtained in the case of surprise. In addition to a greater right-side response, an analogous left-side increase in activity was found for BIS subjects. This effect can be explained by taking into account the emotional valence of surprise, since surprise could be perceived as either a negative or a positive expression. In the present case, the fact that higher BAS subjects did not show a preferred response for surprise, in analogy with happiness, suggests a mainly negative rather than positive valence attribution to this facial pattern.

The main general conclusion may be the broad significance of the BIS/BAS approach in determining subjects' cortical responses as a function of the significance of emotional faces. In considering the effect of emotion type, it is clear that the valence (positive *vs* negative) of faces is not sufficient to explain emotional responses. In fact, among the negatively valenced emotions, sadness did not produce an increased right-side response in BIS subjects; rather there was an equal contribution by the two hemispheres. This interesting effect can be integrated in Gray's model. Accordingly, sadness generated an undifferentiated response by the BIS/BAS, and both cortical sides were implicated in the response to this expression. This points out potential difference in the significance of this expression, and the related emotion in general, within the functional model of emotion perception [80, 87]. Sadness may be a less prominent emotion, since it does not imply a direct and immediate threat to the individual's safety. It may instead be a "secondary" emotion, acquired later in development [88]. In other words, the effect of aversive and negative emotional cues could be greater for unpleasant threatening stimuli, which are generally considered as slightly more arousing for human safety than is the case for less prominent stimuli [89].

References

1. Dimberg U, Öhman A (1996) Behold the wrath: psychophysiological responses to facial stimuli. Motiv Emotion 20:149-182
2. Fernández-Dols JM, Carroll JM (1997) Is the meaning perceived in facial expression independent of its context? In: Russell JA, Fernández-Dols JM (eds) The psychology of facial expression. Cambridge University Press, Cambridge, MA, pp 275-294
3. Caldognetto EM, Cosi P, Drioli C et al (2004) Modifications of phonetic labial targets in emotive speech: effects of the co-production of speech and emotions. Speech Communication. Special Issue: Audio Visual Speech Processing 44:173-185
4. McNeill D (1985) So you think gestures are nonverbal? Psychol Bull 92:350-371
5. Balconi M (2004) Neuropsicologia delle emozioni [Neuropsychology of emotion]. Carocci, Roma
6. Schwarzer T, Leder H (2003) The development of face processing. Hogrefe & Huber, Göttingen
7. Lobaugh NJ, Gibson E, Taylor MJ (2006) Children recruit distinct neural systems for implicit emotional face processing. Neuroreport 17:215-219
8. De Hann M, Pascalis O, Johnson MH (2002) Specialization of neural mechanisms underlying face recognition in human infants. J Cognitive Neurosci 14:199-209
9. Balconi M, Carrera A (2007) Emotional representation in facial expression and script. A comparison between normal and autistic children. Res Dev Disabil 28:409-422
10. Bullock M, Russell JA (1986) Concepts of emotion in developmental psychology. In: Izard CE, Read PB (eds) Measuring emotions in infants and children, Vol. 2. Cambridge University Press, Cambridge, MA, pp 203-237
11. Widen SC, Russell JA (2003) A closer look at preschoolers' freely produced labels for facial expressions. Dev Psychol 39:114-128
12. Davidson R J, Ekman P, Saron CD et al (1990) Approach-withdrawal and cerebral asymmetry: emotional expression and brain physiology I. J Pers Soc Psychol 58:330-341
13. Cacioppo JT, Berntson GG (1994) Relationships between and evaluative space: a critical review with emphasis on the separability of positive and negative substrates. Psychol Bull 115:401-423
14. Allen JJB, Kline JP (2004) Frontal EEG asymmetry, emotion, and psychopathology: the first, and the next 25 years. Biol Psychol 67:1-5
15. Russell J (1980) A circumplex model of affect. J Pers Soc Psychol 39:1161-1178

16. Bradley MM, Lang PJ (2007) The International Affective Picture System (IAPS) in the study of emotion and attention. In: Coan JA, Allen JJB (eds) Handbook of emotion elicitation and assessment. Oxford University Press, Oxford, pp 38-395
17. Cuthbert BN, Schupp HT, Bradley MM et al (2000) Brain potentials in affective picture processing: covariation with autonomic arousal and affective report. Biol Psychol 62:95-111
18. Lang PJ, Greenwald MK, Bradley MM, Hamm AO (1993) Looking at pictures: affective, facial, visceral, and behavioral reactions. Psychophysiol 30:261-273
19. Everhart DE, Harrison DW (2000) Facial affect perception in anxious and nonanxious men without depression. Psychobiol 28:90-98
20. Heller W (1993) Neuropsychological mechanisms of individual differences in emotion, personality, and arousal. Neuropsychol 7:476-489
21. Gray JA (1981) A critique of Eysenck's theory of personality. In: Eysenck HJ (ed) A model for personality. Springer, Berlin, pp 246-277
22. Carver CS, White TL (1994) Behavioral inhibition, behavioral activation, and affective responses to impending reward and punishment: the BIS/BAS Scales. J Pers Soc Psychol 67:319-333
23. Gray JA (1990) Brain systems that mediate both emotion and cognition. Cognition Emotion 4:269-288
24. Fowles DC (1980) The three arousal model: implications of Gray's two-factor learning theory for heart rate, electrodermal activity, and psychopathy. Psychophysiology 17:87-104
25. Gray JA (1982) The neuropsychology of anxiety: an inquiry into the functions of the septo-hippocampal system. Oxford University Press, New York
26. Gray JA, McNaughton N (2000) The neuropsychology of anxiety: an enquiry into the functions of the septo-hippocampal system. Oxford University Press, Oxford
27. Tomarken AJ, Davidson RJ, Wheeler RE, Kinney L (1992) Psychometric properties of resting anterior EEG asymmetry: temporal stability and internal consistency. Psychophysiology 29:576-559
28. Harmon-Jones E, Sigelman J (2001) State anger and prefrontal brain activity: evidence that insult-related relative left-prefrontal activation is associated with experienced anger and aggression. J Pers Soc Psychol 80:797-803
29. Corr PJ (2002) J.A. Gray's reinforcement sensitivity theory and frustrative nonreward: a theoretical note on expectancies in reactions to rewarding stimuli. Pers Indiv Differ 32:1247-1253
30. Yu AJ, Dayan P (2005) Uncertainty, neuromodulation, and attention. Neuron 46:681-69
31. Quay HC (1988) Attention deficit disorder and the behavioral inhibition system: the relevance of the neuropsychological theory of Jeffrey A. Gray. In: Bloomingdale LM, Sergeant JA (eds) Attention deficit disorder: criteria, cognition, intervention. Pergamon, Oxford, pp 117-125
32. Newman JP, MacCoon DG, Vaughn LJ, Sadeh N (2005) Validating a distinction between primary and secondary psychopathy with measures of Gray's BIS and BAS Constructs. J Abnorm Psychol 114:319-323
33. Keil A, Bradley MM, Hauk O et al (2002) Large-scale neural correlates of affective picture processing. Psychophysiol 39:641-649
34. Aftanas L, Varlamov A, Pavlov S et al (2002) Time-dependent cortical asymmetries induced by emotional arousal: EEG analysis of event-related synchronization and desynchronization in individually defined frequency bands. Int J Psychophysiol 44:67-82
35. Balconi M, Lucchiari C (2007) Encoding of emotional facial expressions in direct and incidental tasks: two event-related potentials studies. Aust J Psychol 59:13-23
36. Basąr E, Demiralp T, Schürmann M et al (1999) Oscillatory brain dynamics, wavelet analysis, and cognition. Brain Lang 66:146-183

11

37. Krause CM, Viemerö V, Rosenqvist A et al (2000) Relative electroencephalographic desyncronization and syncronization in humans to emotional film content: an analysis of the 4-6, 6-8, 8-10 and 10-12 Hz frequency bands. Neurosci Letters 286:9-12
38. Balconi M, Lucchiari C (2007) Event-related oscillations (EROs) and eventrelated potentials (ERPs) comparison in facial expression recognition. J Neuropsychol 1:283-294
39. Knyazev GG (2007) Motivation, emotion, and their inhibitory control mirrored in brain oscillations. Neurosci Biobehav R 31:377-395
40. Ward LM (2003) Synchronous neural oscillations and cognitive processes. Trends Cognitive Sci 7:553-559.
41. Balconi M, Lucchiari C (2008) Consciousness and arousal effects on emotional face processing as revealed by brain oscillations. A gamma band analysis. Int J Psychophysiol 67:41-46
42. Güntekin B, Basąr E (2007) Emotional face expressions are differentiated with brain oscillations. Int J Psychophysiol 64:91-100
43. Harmon-Jones E, Allen JJB (1997) Behavioral activation sensitivity and resting frontal EEG asymmetry: covariation of putative indicators related to risk for mood disorders. J Abnorm Psychol 106:159-163.
44. Hewig J, Hagemann D, Seifert J et al (2006) The relation of cortical activity and BIS/BAS on the trait level. Biol Psychol 71:42-53
45. Knyazev GG, Slobodskoj-Plusnin JY (2007) Behavioural approach system as a moderator of emotional arousal elicited by reward and punishment cues. Pers Individ Differ 42:49-59
46. Coan JA, Allen JJB (2003) Frontal EEG asymmetry and the behavioral activation and inhibition systems. Psychophysiology 40:106-114
47. Sutton S K, Davidson RJ (1997) Prefrontal brain asymmetry: a biological substrate of the behavioral approach and inhibition systems. Psychol Sci, 8:204-210
48. Davidson RJ, Henriques J (2000) Regional brain function in sadness and depression. Oxford University Press, New York
49. Waldstein SR, Kop WJ, Schmidt LA et al (2000) Frontal electrocortical and cardiovascular reactivity during happiness and anger. Biol Psychol 55:3-23
50. Wheeler RE, Davidson RJ, Tomarken AJ (1993) Frontal brain asymmetry and emotional reactivity: a biological substrate of affective style. Psychophysiology 30:82-89
51. Harmon-Jones E, Sigelman JD, Bohlig A, Harmon-Jones C (2003) Anger, coping, and frontal cortical activity: the effect of coping potential on anger-induced left-frontal activity. Cogn Em 17:1-24
52. Aftanas L, Varlamov A, Pavlov S et al (2001) Event-related synchronization and desynchronization during affective processing: emergence of valence-related time-dependent hemispheric asymmetries in theta and upper alpha band. Int J Neurosci 110:197-219
53. Karakas S, Erzengin OU, Basąr EA (2000) A new strategy involving multiple cognitive paradigms demonstrates that ERP components are determined by the superposition of oscillatory responses. Clinical Neurophysiol 111:1719-1732
54. Iragui VJ, Kutas M, Mitchiner MR, Hillyard SAE (1993) Effects of aging on event-related brain potentials and reaction times in an auditory oddball task. Psychophysiology 30:10-22
55. Basąr E, Basar-Eroglu C, Karakas S, Schürmann M (2000) Brain oscillations in perception and memory. Int J Psychophysiol. Special Issue: Proceedings of the 9th World Congress of the International Organization of Psychophysiology (IOP) 35:95-124.
56. Krause CM (2003) Brain electric oscillations and cognitive processes. In: Hugdahl K (ed) Experimental methods in neuropsychology. Kluwer, New York, pp 11-130
57. Sato W, Takanori K, Sakiko Y, Michikazu M (2001) Emotional expression boosts early visual processing of the face: ERP reecording and its decomposition by independent component analysis. Neuroreport 12:709-714

58. Lang PJ, Bradley MM, Cuthbert BN (1997) Motivated attention: affect, activation, and action. In: Lang PJ, Simons RF, Balaban M (eds) Attention and orienting: sensory and motivational processes, Erlbaum, Mahwah, pp 97-135
59. Balconi M, Pozzoli U (2003) Face-selective processing and the effect of pleasant and unpleasant emotional expressions on ERP correlates. Int J Psychophysiol 49:67-74
60. Ladavas E, Umiltà C, Ricci-Bitti PE (1980) Evidence for sex differences in right-hemisphere dominance for emotions. Giornale Italiano di Psicologia 7:121-127.
61. Safer MA, Leventhal H (1977) Ear differences in evaluating emotional tones of voice and verbal content. J Exp Psychol Human 3:75-82
62. Etcoff N (1989) Asymmetries in recognition of emotion. In: Boller F, Grafman J (eds) Handbook of neuropsychology. Elsevier, New York, pp 363-382
63. Borod JC (1993) Cerebral mechanisms underlying facial, prosodic, and lexical emotional expression: a review of neuropsychological studies and methodological issues. Neuropsychology 7:445-463
64. Root JC, Wong PS, Kinsbourne M (2006) Left hemisphere specialization for response to positive emotional expressions: a divided output methodology. Emotion 6:473-483
65. Adolphs R, Damasio H, Tranel D, Damasio AR (1996) Cortical systems for the recognition of emotion in facial expressions. J Neurosci 16:7678-7687
66. Ahern GL, Schomer DL, Kleefield J, Blume H (1991) Right hemisphere advantage for evaluating emotional facial expressions. Cortex 27:193-202
67. Sato W, Kochiyama T, Yoshikawa S et al (2004) Enhanced neural activity in response to dynamic facial expressions of emotion: an fMRI study. Cognitive Brain Res 20:81-91
68. Vanderploeg RD, Brown WS, Marsh JT (1987) Judgments of emotion in words and faces: ERP correlates. Int J Psychophysiol 5:193-205
69. Borod JC, Haywood CS, Koff E (1997) Neuropsychological aspects of facial asymmetry during emotional expression: a review of the normal adult literature. Neuropsychol Rev 7:41-60
70. Gainotti G (1972) Emotional behavior and hemispheric side of the lesion. Cortex 8:41-55
71. Everhart DE, Carpenter MD, Carmona JE et al (2003) Adult sex-related P300 differences during the perception of emotional prosody and facial affect. Psychophysiology 40:S39
72. Silberman EK, Weingartner H (1986) Hemispheric lateralization of functions related to emotion. Brain Cognition 5:322-353
73. Reuter-Lorenz P A, Givis RP, Moscovitch M (1983) Hemispheric specialization and the perception of emotion: evidence from right-handers and from inverted and non-inverted left-handers. Neuropsychologia 21:687-692
74. Everhart DE, Harrison DW (2000) Facial affect perception in anxious and nonanxious men without depression. Psychobiol 28:90-98
75. Schellberg D, Besthorn C, Pfleger W, Gasser T (1993) Emotional activation and topographic EEG band power. J Psychophysiol 7:24-33
76. Davidson RJ, Fox NA (1982) Asymmetrical brain activity discriminates between positive and negative affective stimuli in human infants. Science 218:1235-1237
77. Waldstein SR, Kop WJ, Schmidt LA et al (2000) Frontal electrocortical and cardiovascular reactivity during happiness and anger. Biol Psychol 55:3-23
78. Coan JA, Allen JJB, Harmon-Jones E (2001) Voluntary facial expression and hemispheric asymmetry over the frontal cortex. Psychophysiol 38:912-925
79. Harmon-Jones E, Allen JJB (1998) Anger and frontal brain activity: EEG asymmetry consistent with approach motivation despite negative affective valence. J Pers Soc Psychol 74:1310-1316
80. Frijda NH (1994) Emotions are functional, most of the time. In: Ekman P, Davidson RJ (eds) The nature of emotion: fundamental questions. Oxford University Press, New York, pp 112-122
81. Frijda NH, Kuipers P, Terschure E (1989) Relations among emotion, appraisal, and emotional action readiness. J Pers Soc Psychol 57:212-228

82. Balconi M, Mazza G (2008) Lateralisation effect in comprehension of emotional facial expression: a comparison between EEG alpha band power and behavioural inhibition (BIS) and activation (BAS) systems. Laterality 17:1-24
83. Junghöfer M, Bradley MM, Elbert T R, Lang PJ (2001) Fleeting images: a new look at early emotion discrimination. Psychophysiology 38:175-178
84. Harmon-Jones E, Sigelman JD, Bohlig A, Harmon-Jones C (2003) Anger, coping, and frontal cortical activity: the effect of coping potential on anger-induced left-frontal activity. Cognition Emotion 17:1-24
85. Gable S L, Reis HT, Elliot AJ (2000) Behavioral activation and inhibition in everyday life. J Pers Soc Psychol 78:1135-1149
86. Sutton SK, Davidson RJ (2000) Prefrontal brain electrical asymmetry predicts the evaluation of affective stimuli. Neuropsychologia 38:1723-1733
87. Hamm AO, Schupp HT, Weike AI (2003) Motivational organization of emotions: autonomic change, cortical response and reflex modulation. In: Davidson RJ, Scherer KR, Goldsmith HH (eds) Handbook of affective science. Oxford University Press, New York, pp 187-212
88. Russell JA (2003) Core affect and the psychological construction of emotion. Psychol Rev 110:145-172
89. Wild B, Erb M, Bartels M (2001) Are emotions contagious? Evoked emotions while viewing emotionally expressive faces: quality, quantity, time course and gender differences. Psychiat Res 102:109-124

Subject Index

MIX
Papier aus verantwortungsvollen Quellen
Paper from responsible sources
FSC® C105338

If you have any concerns about our products,
you can contact us on
ProductSafety@springernature.com

In case Publisher is established outside the EU,
the EU authorized representative is:
Springer Nature Customer Service Center GmbH
Europaplatz 3, 69115 Heidelberg, Germany

Printed by Libri Plureos GmbH
in Hamburg, Germany